Look Out —
Minibeasts About!

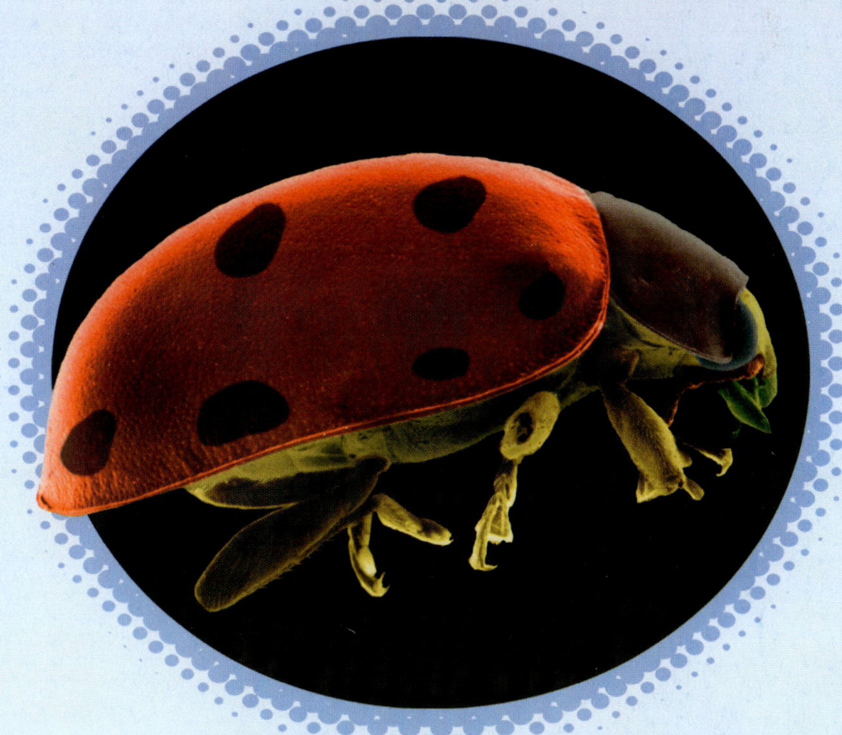

Haydn Middleton

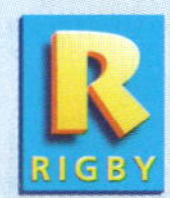

Contents

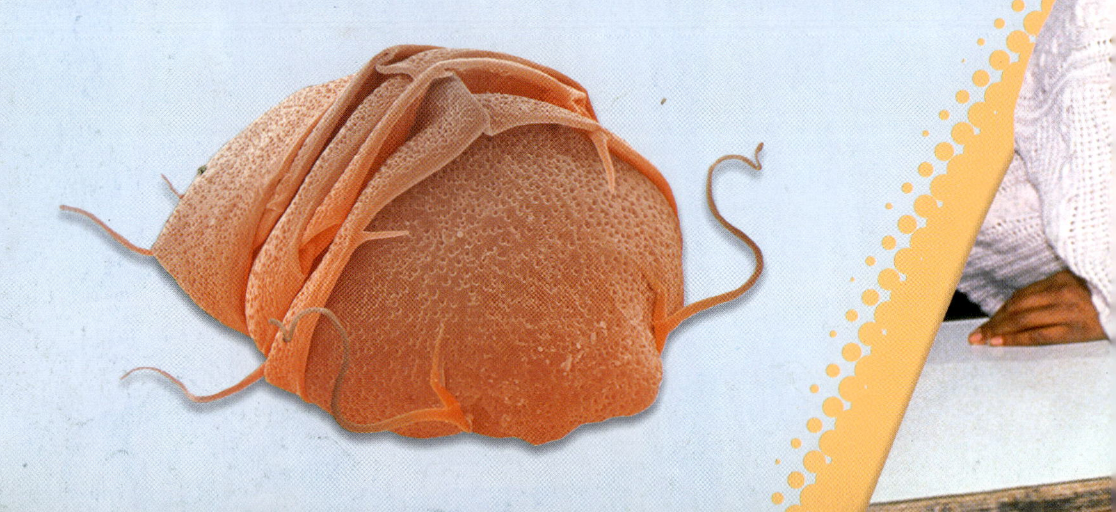

1 Tiny is Amazing

Some of them live in your garden. Some of them live in your home. Some of them live on you! What are they? They are minibeasts! Some of them are so tiny that you can only see them with a microscope.

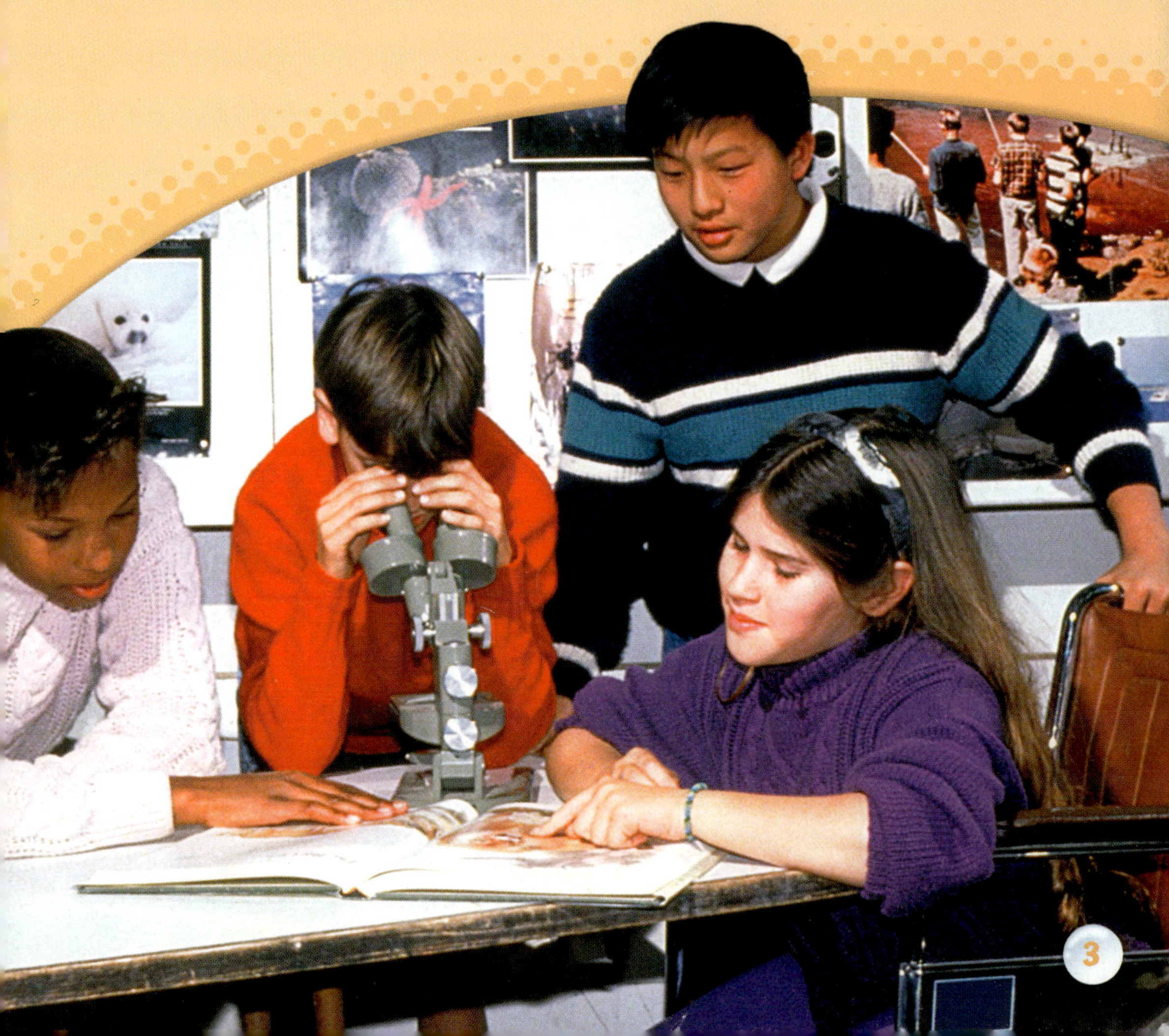

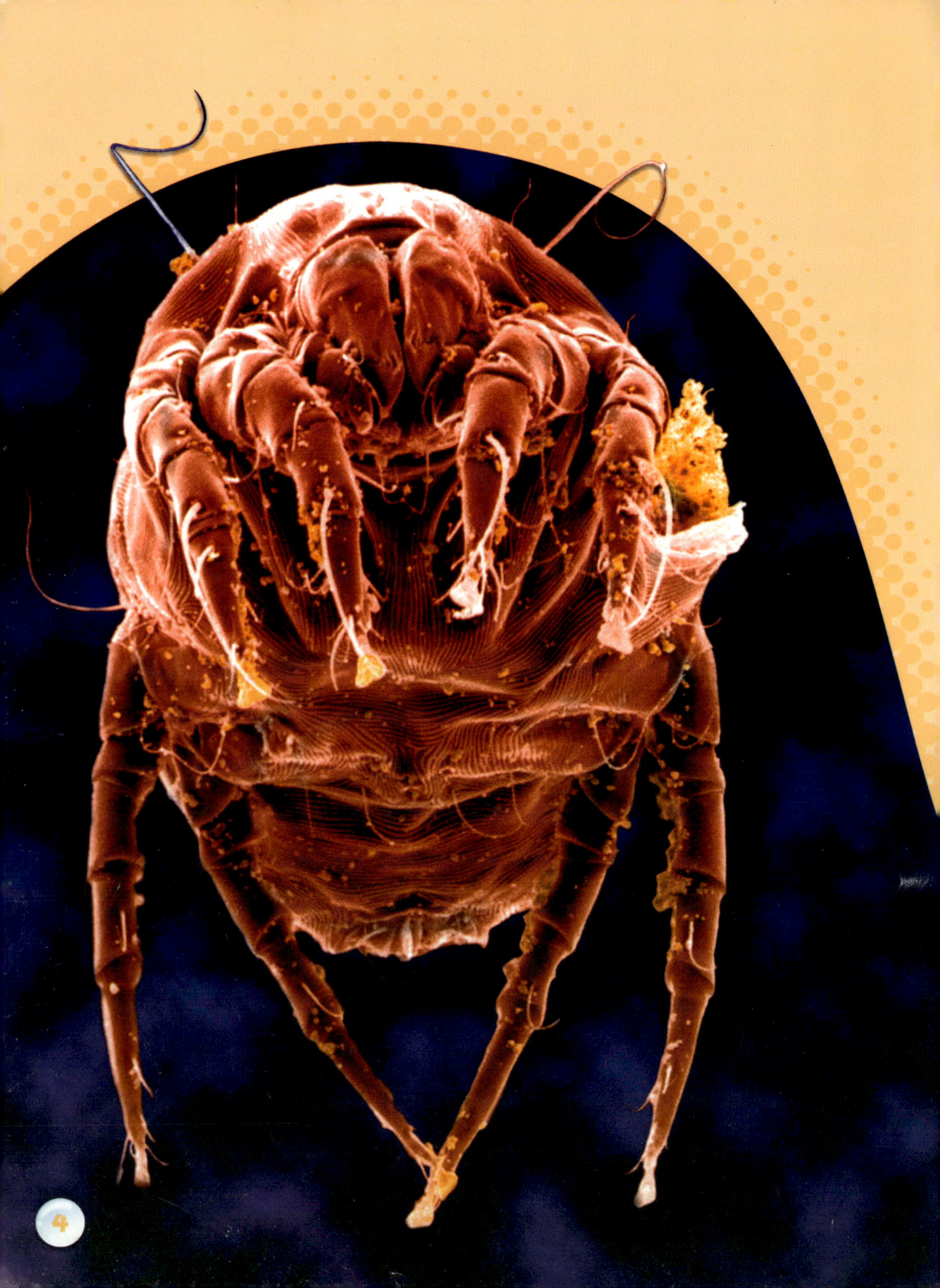

This minibeast lives in your bed. Do you know what it is? It is a dust mite. But it is not the only dust mite that lives in your bed. There are more than a million of them!

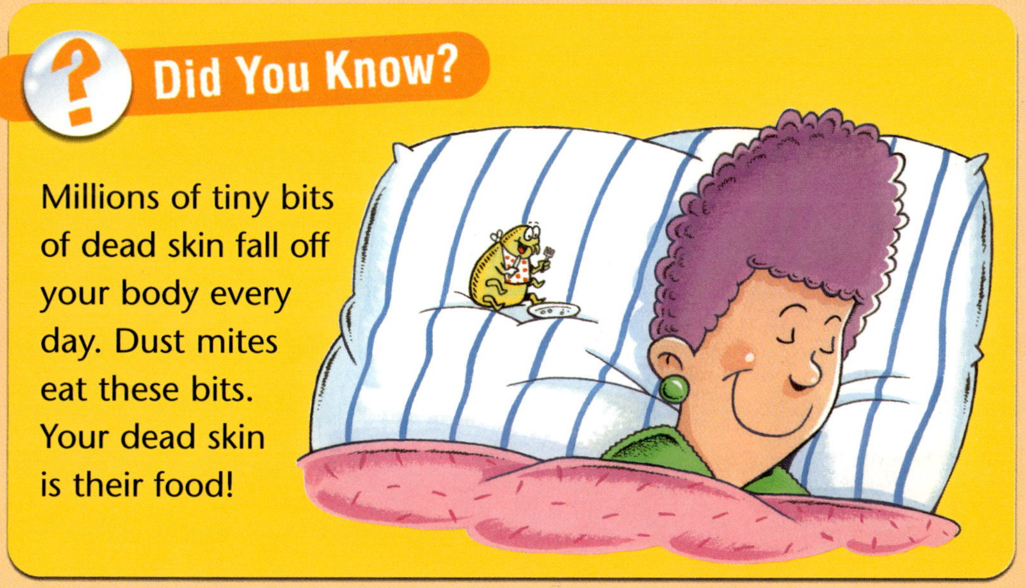

In this book, you will meet many more minibeasts. They look amazing. They do amazing things. They live in amazing places.

2 Minibeasts in the Air

The hoverfly is too tiny to see, but you can hear it. It flies very fast. It flaps its wings a thousand times every second! This makes a humming sound.

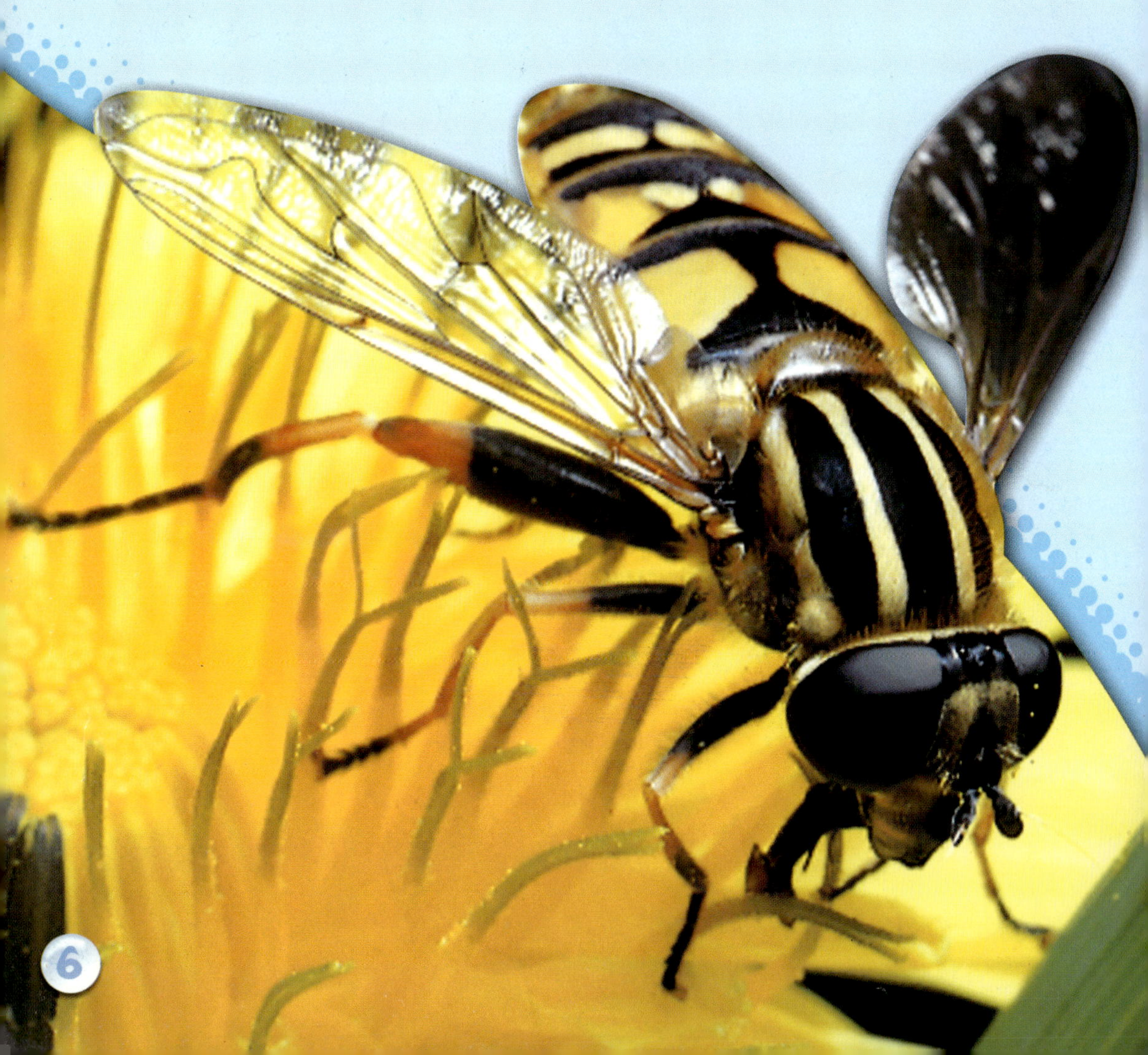

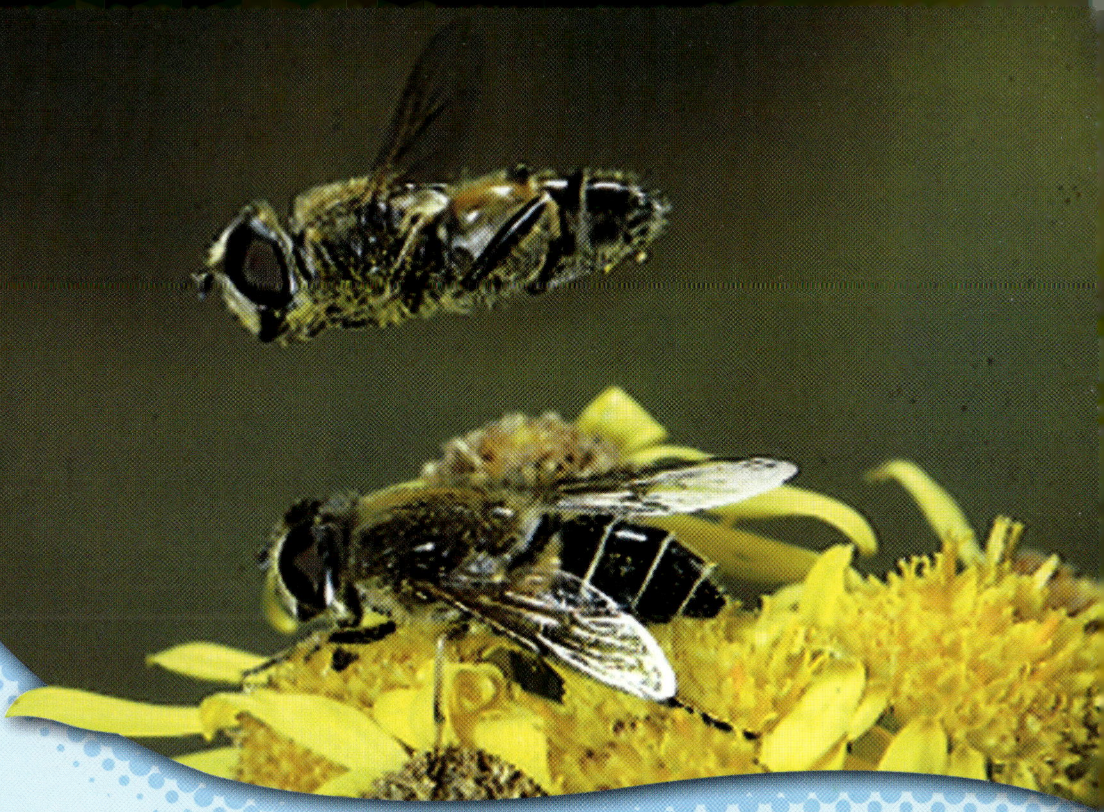

The hoverfly can fly back and forth and sideways.
It can even stay still in mid-air. The male hoverfly
does this to show off around the female hoverfly!

Did You Know?

One kind of fly lays its eggs in
a sheep's nose! It is called the
sheep nostril fly.

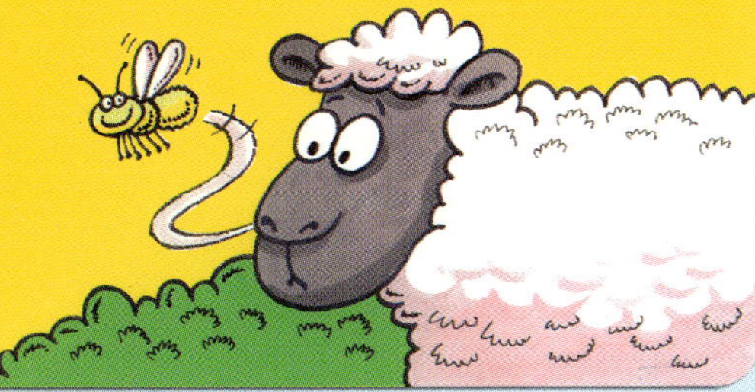

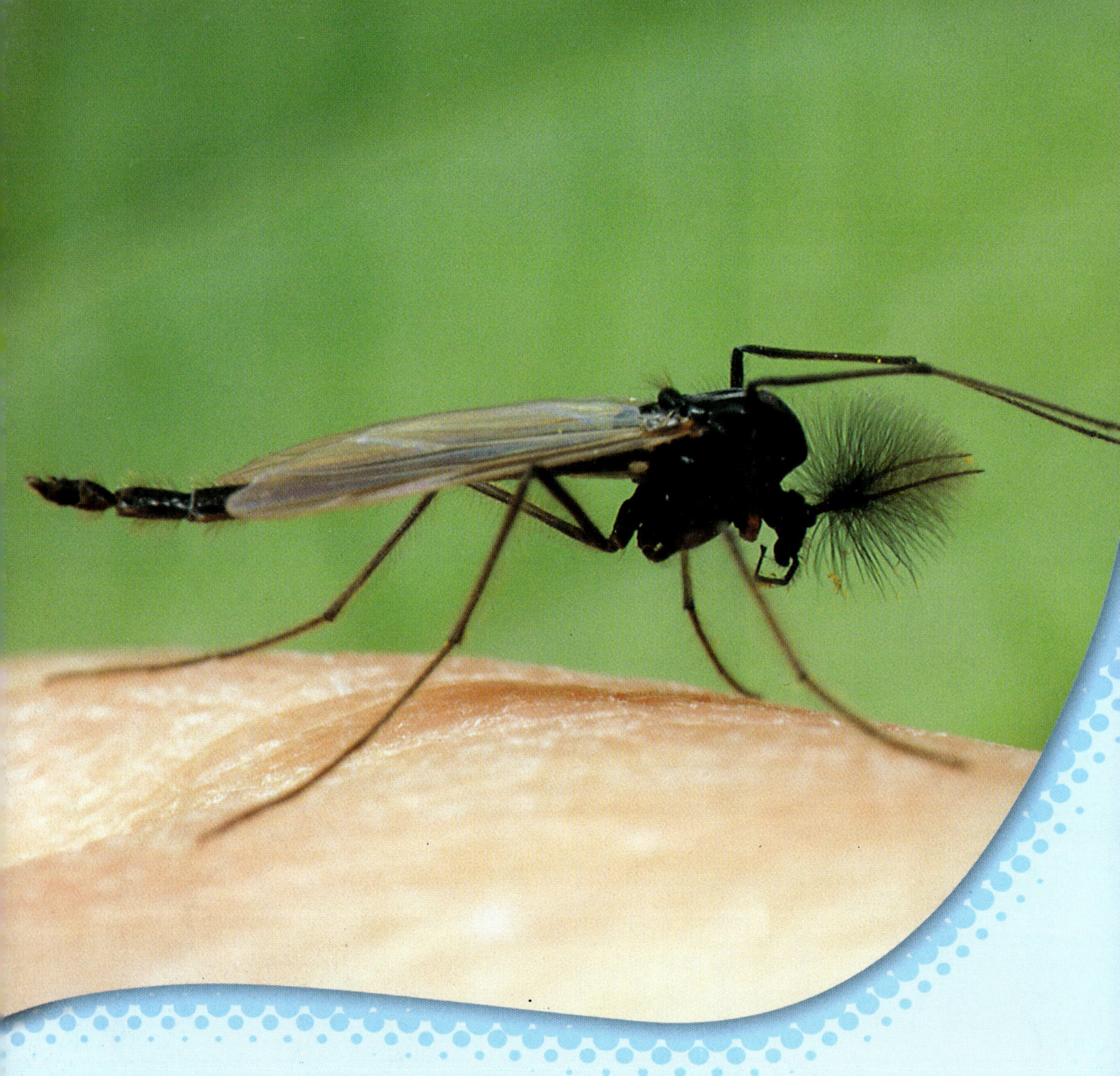

A midge is a busy minibeast. Midges bite people
and suck out their blood. But they don't bite just
anyone. They have feelers on their head that smell
people's sweat. If the sweat smells right, the midge
will bite!

Midges might bite you, but thrips get together and crawl over you. Thrips are minibeasts with wings. They float in the air. Before a storm, thrips group together. Then they fly onto people and crawl all over them! A group of thrips is called a swarm.

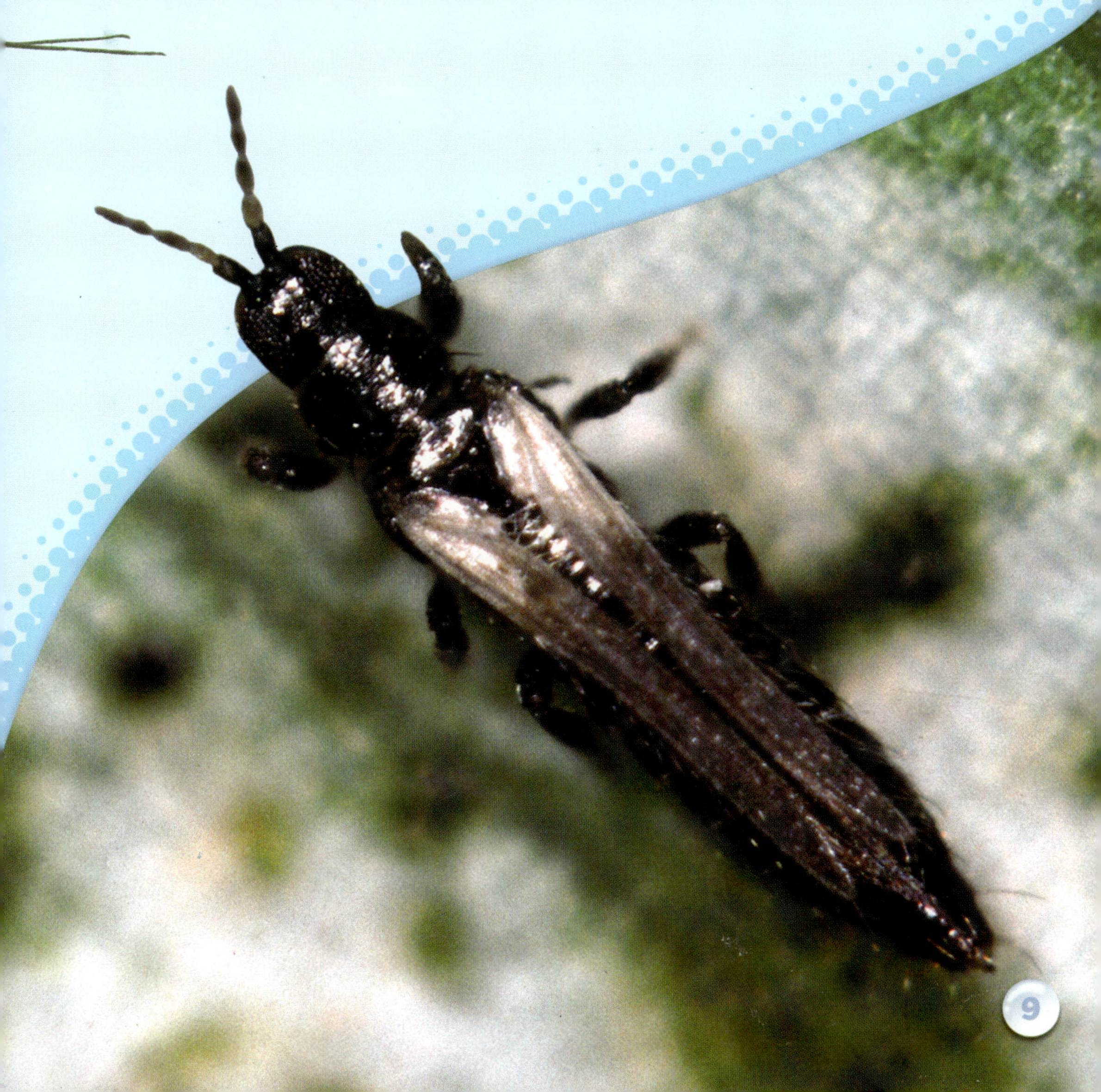

3 Minibeasts on Land

Long ago, most minibeasts lived in water. Then some minibeasts started to live on land. The springtail was one of the first to live on land and there are still springtails on Earth today!

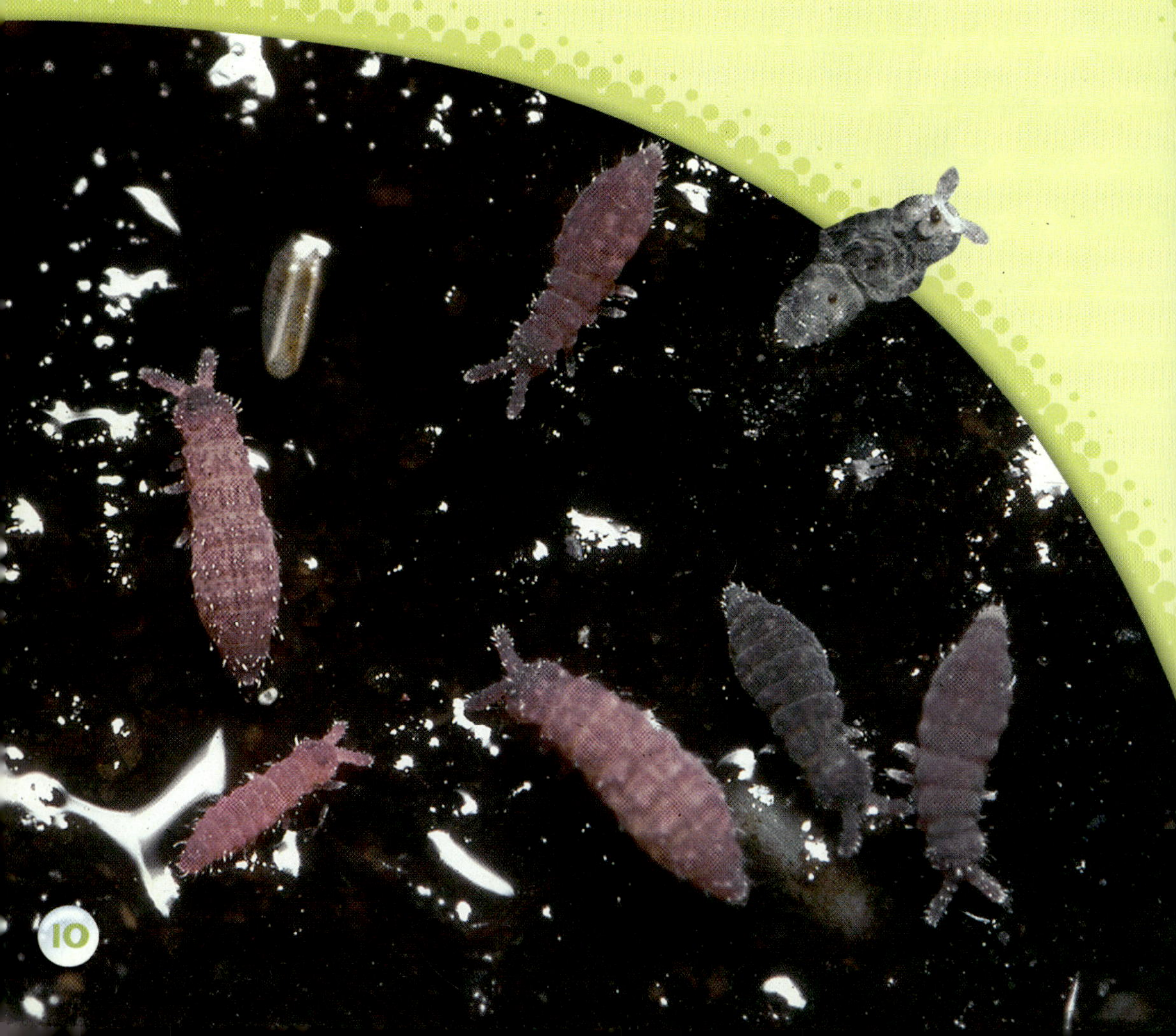

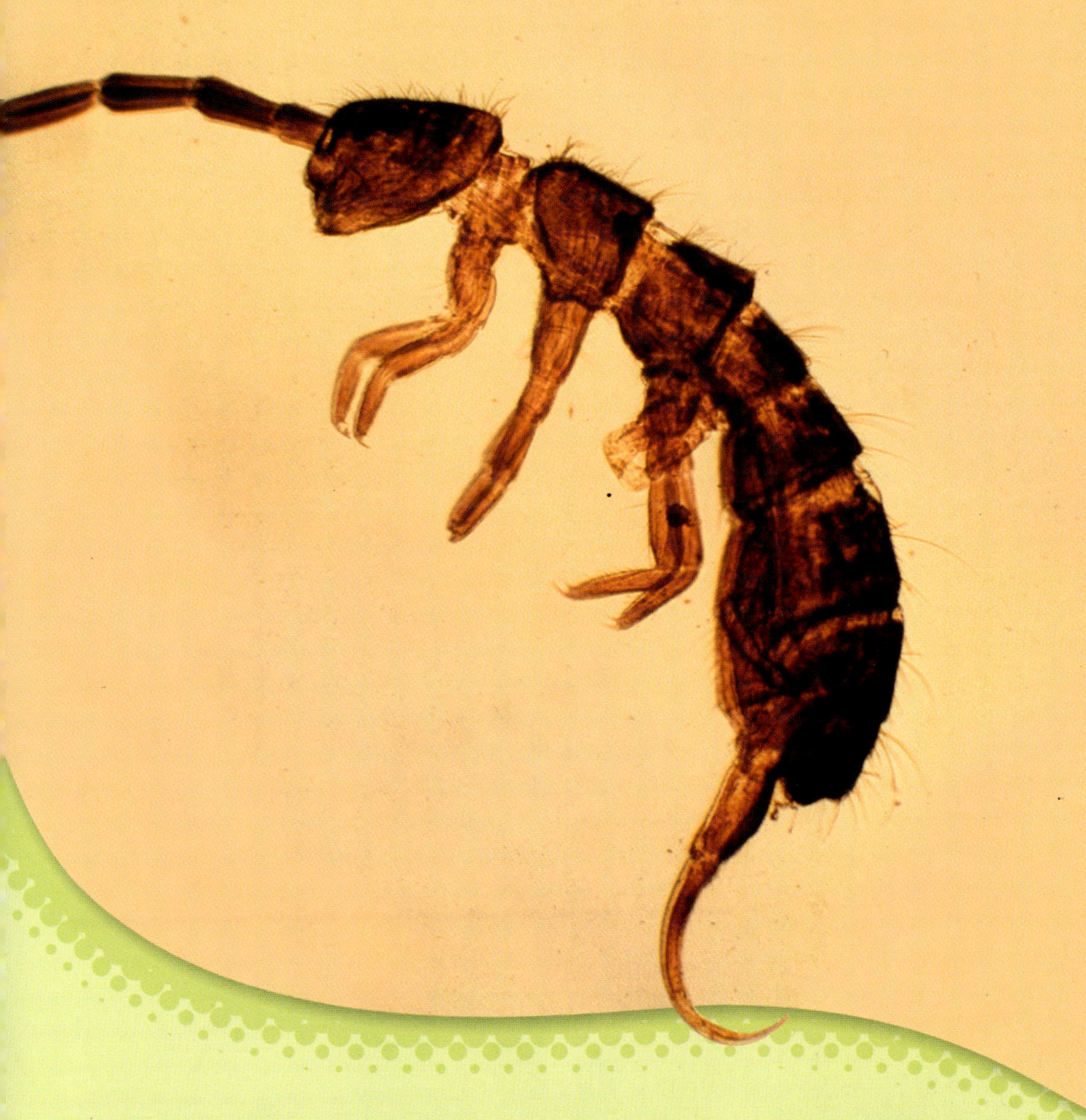

A springtail has a long tail tucked under its body. It pushes its tail out to jump up in the air. Springtails live in damp earth or wet places indoors. They like to eat dead plants.

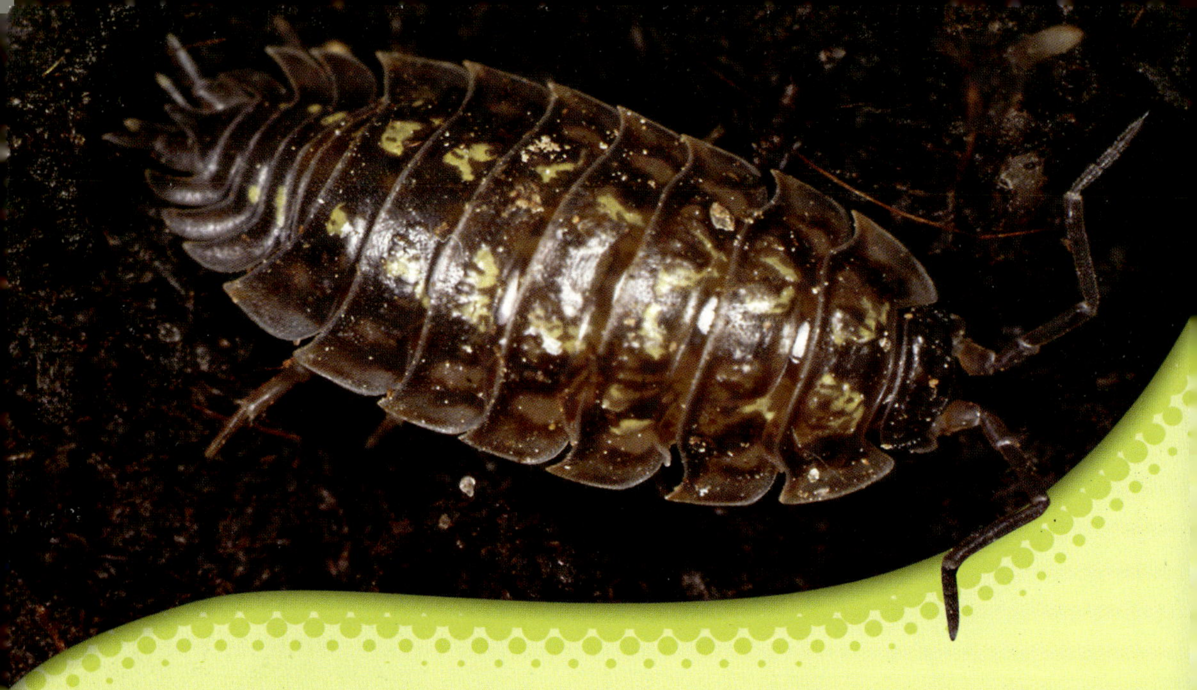

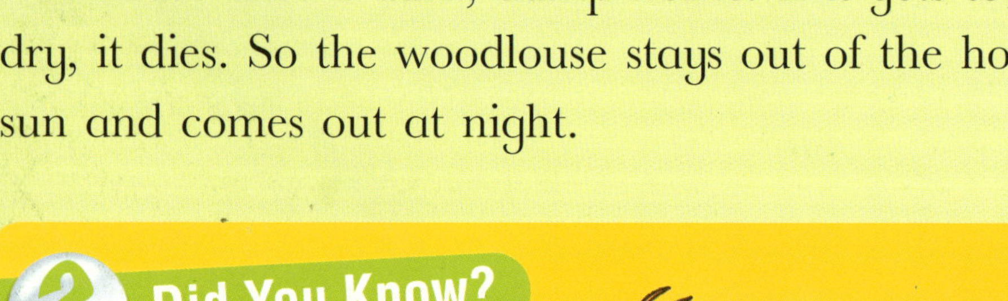

We like our home to be bright and dry. A woodlouse likes a dark, damp home. If it gets too dry, it dies. So the woodlouse stays out of the hot sun and comes out at night.

Did You Know?

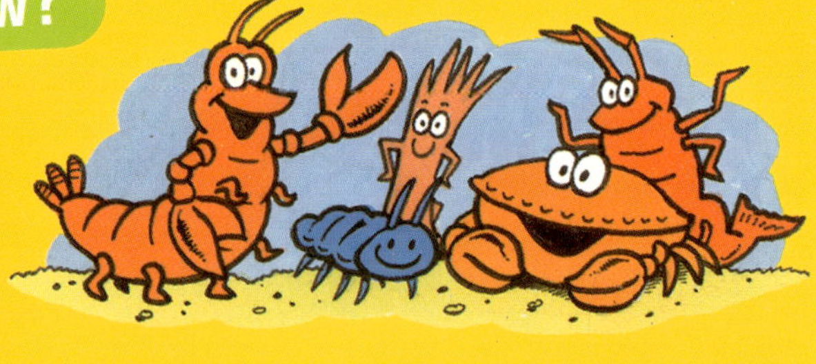

The woodlouse belongs to the crab and lobster family! Most members of this family live in the water and breathe with gills. The woodlouse breathes with gills too! The gills must stay damp, or they do not work.

Baby woodlice hatch from eggs. Then they live with their mother. Most minibeasts don't usually see their mother. The mother just lays her eggs and moves on. Woodlouse mothers stay around!

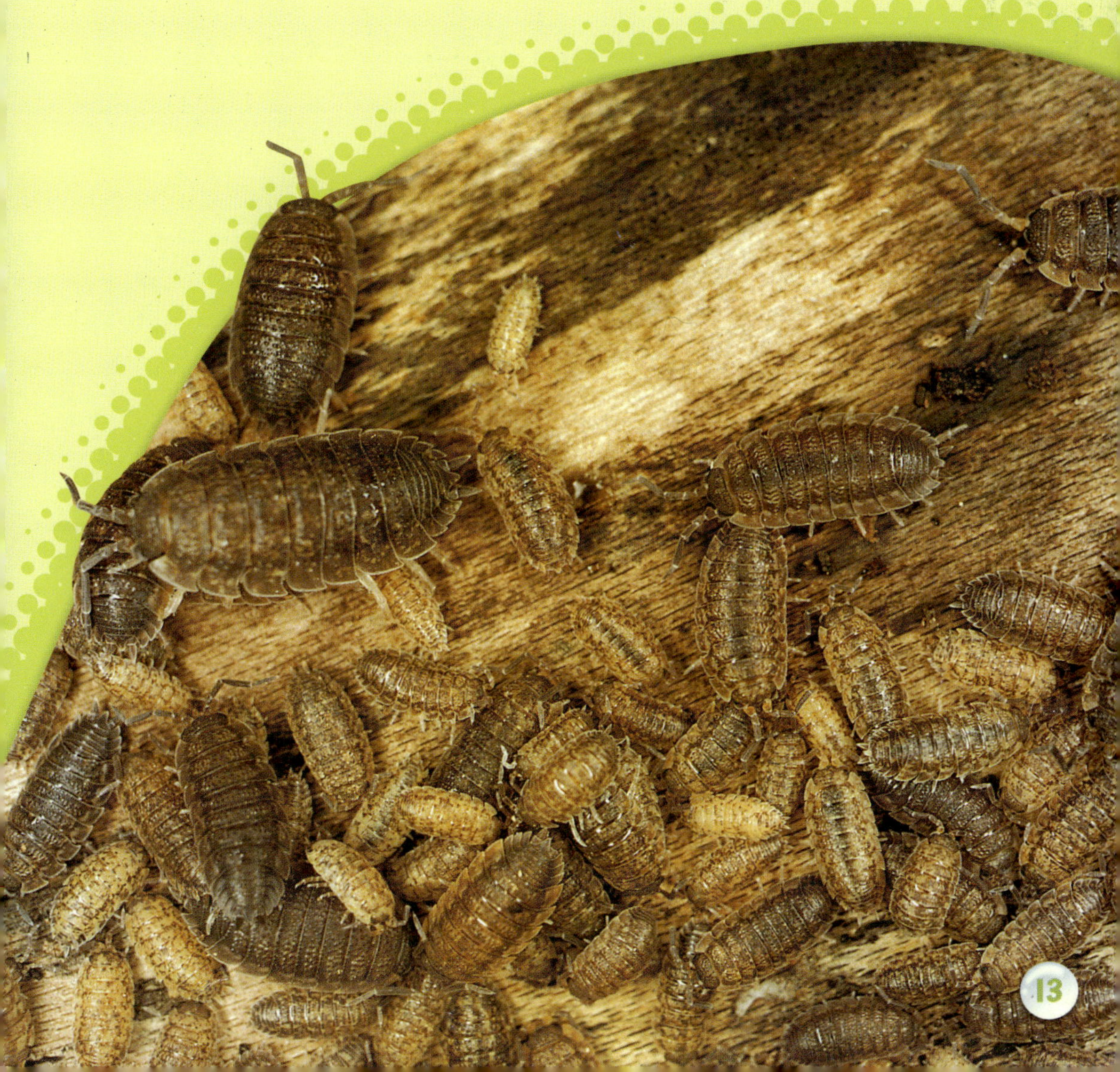

Aphids are tiny garden bugs. They are sometimes called greenflies. Aphids feed on something called sap. Sap is the juice in flowers and plants. Aphids get together in groups that eat up farm plants.

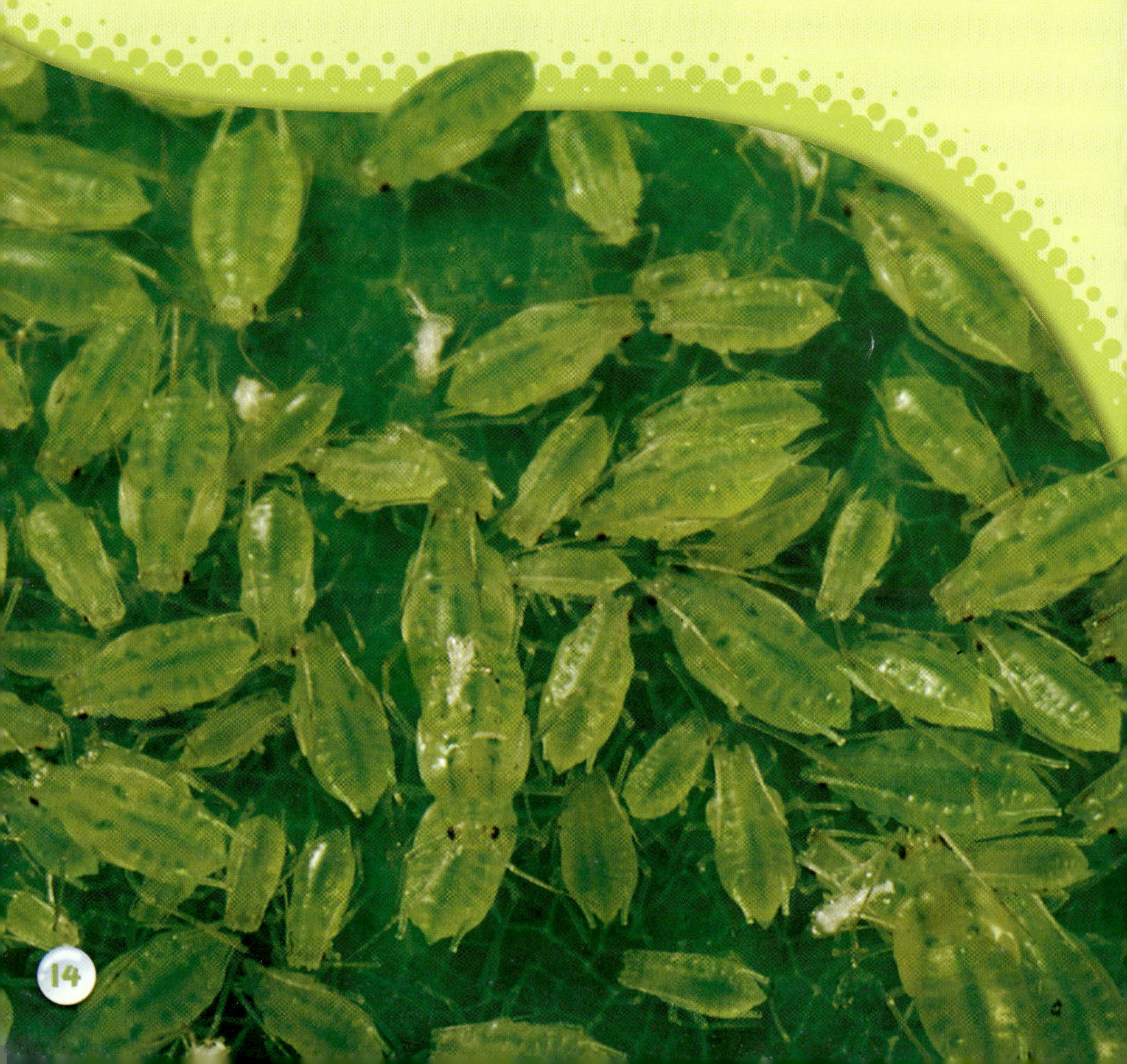

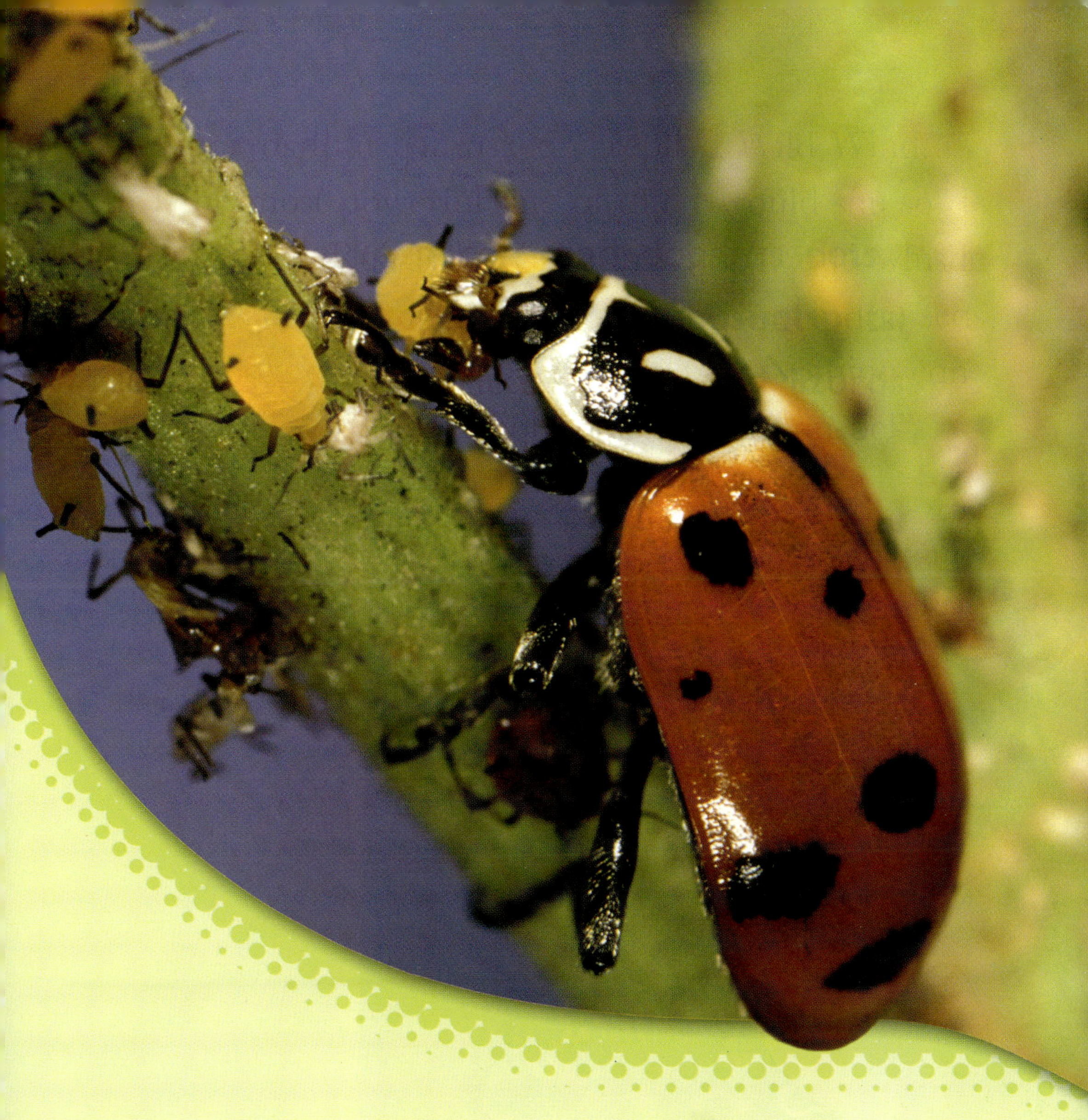

Millions and millions of aphids are born every year. But millions of them die every year too because other bugs like to eat them. A ladybird can eat more than 100 aphids in one day!

4 Minibeasts in Water

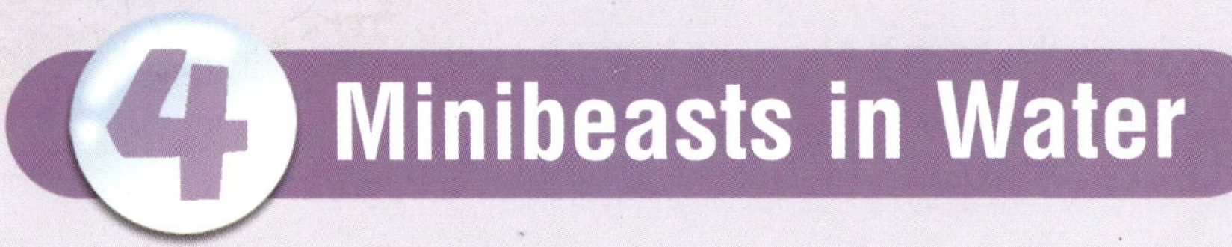

Water bears live in or around ponds. They can be smaller than the dot on an i. They eat minibeasts that are even smaller than they are!

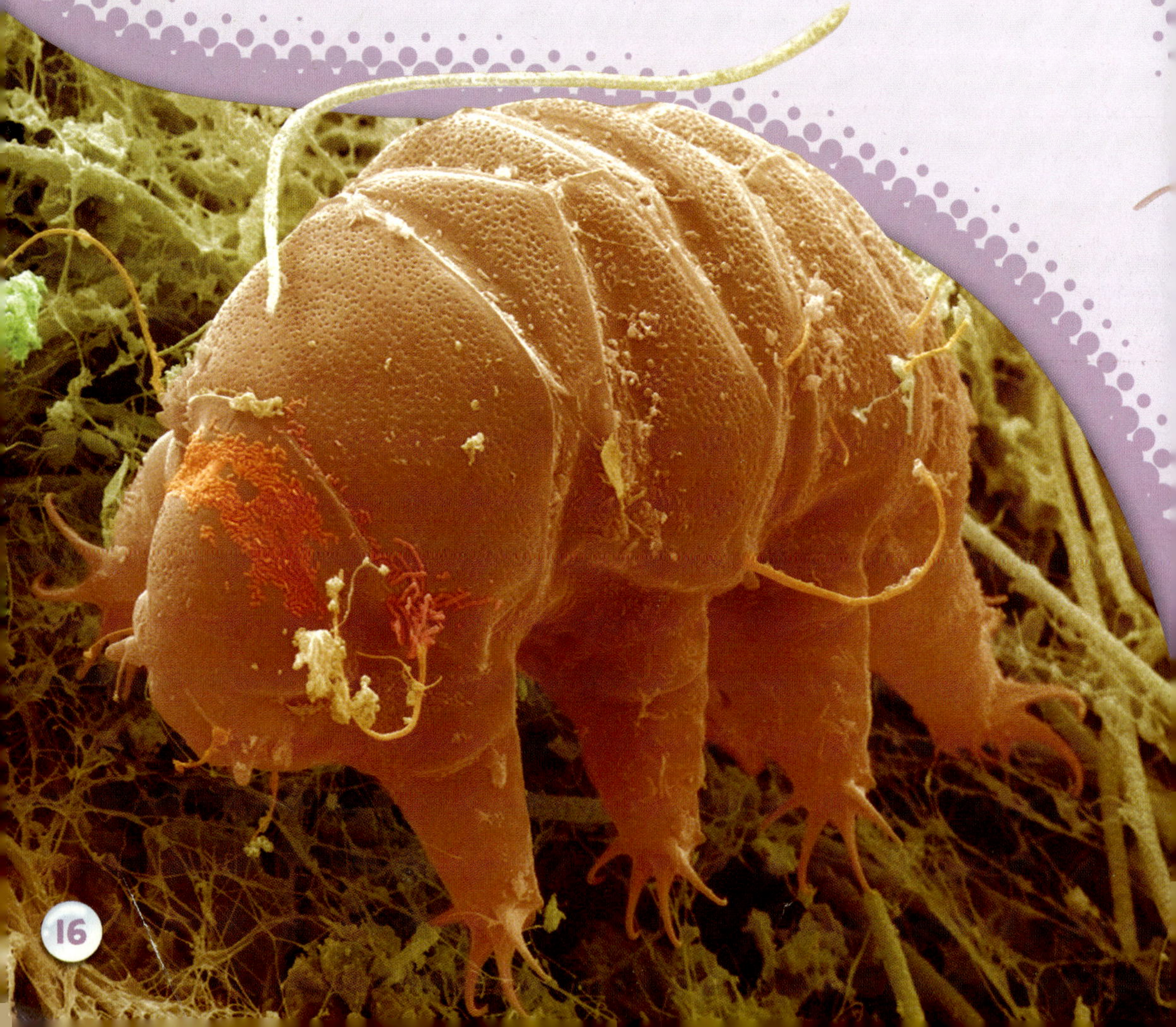

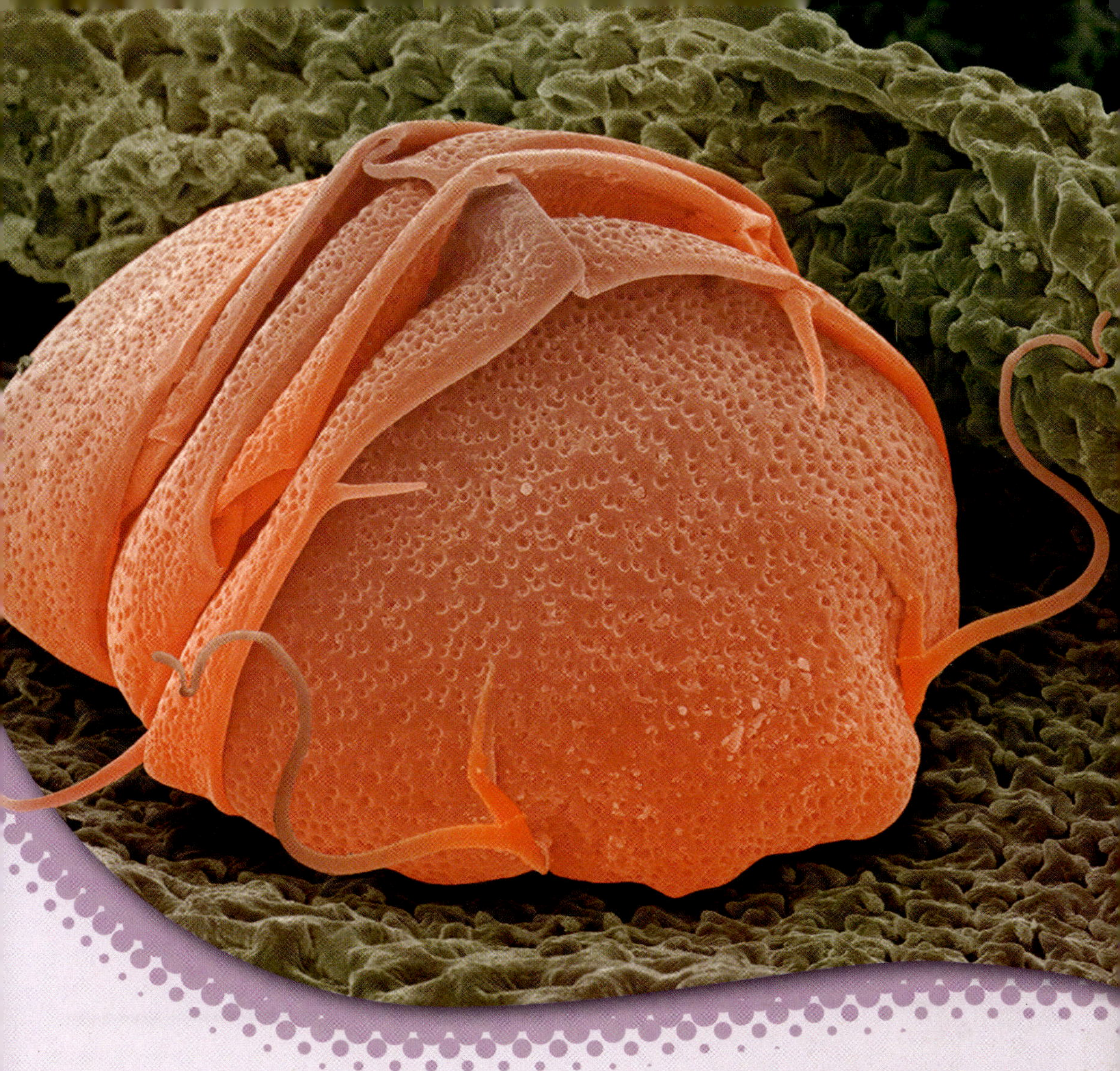

A water bear likes wet or damp places best.
When it gets dry, it changes. It gets smaller and
does not move. It stays small and still for a long
time. When it gets wet again, it gets bigger and
comes back to life!

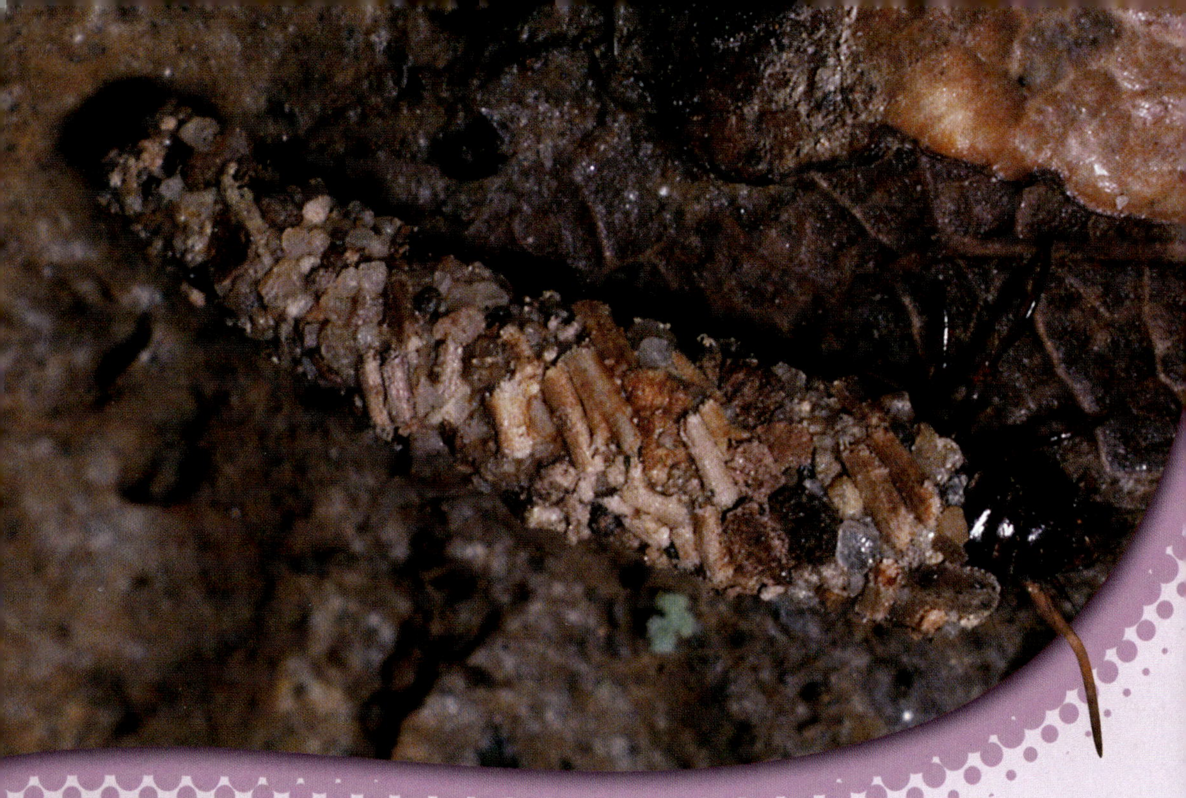

Some minibeasts grow up in the water but then live on land. One kind of fly grows up in a pond. When it is young, it looks like a worm. It is called a larva.

The larva makes a body case to protect itself. It makes the case with bits of dirt and plants. Then it moves around the pond inside the body case.

When the larva is grown up, it leaves the water. It has grown wings and can fly. It has become a minibeast called a caddis-fly.

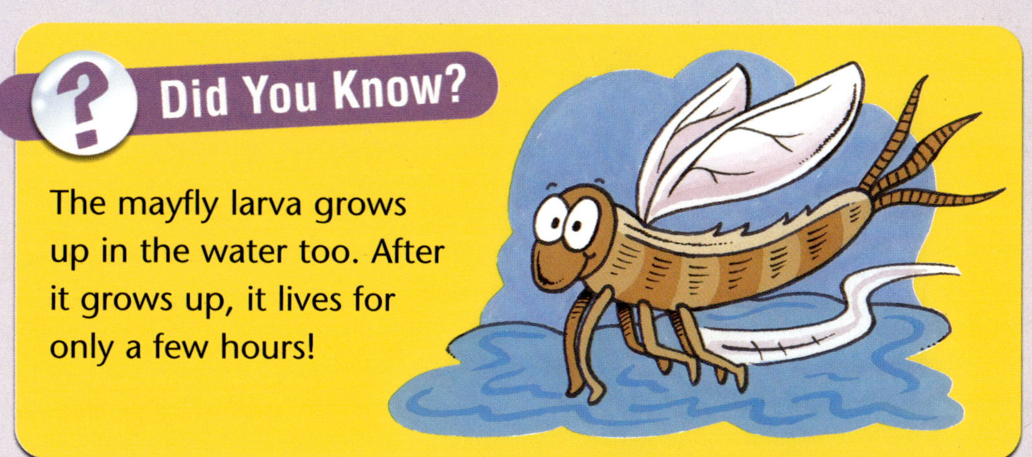

? Did You Know?

The mayfly larva grows up in the water too. After it grows up, it lives for only a few hours!

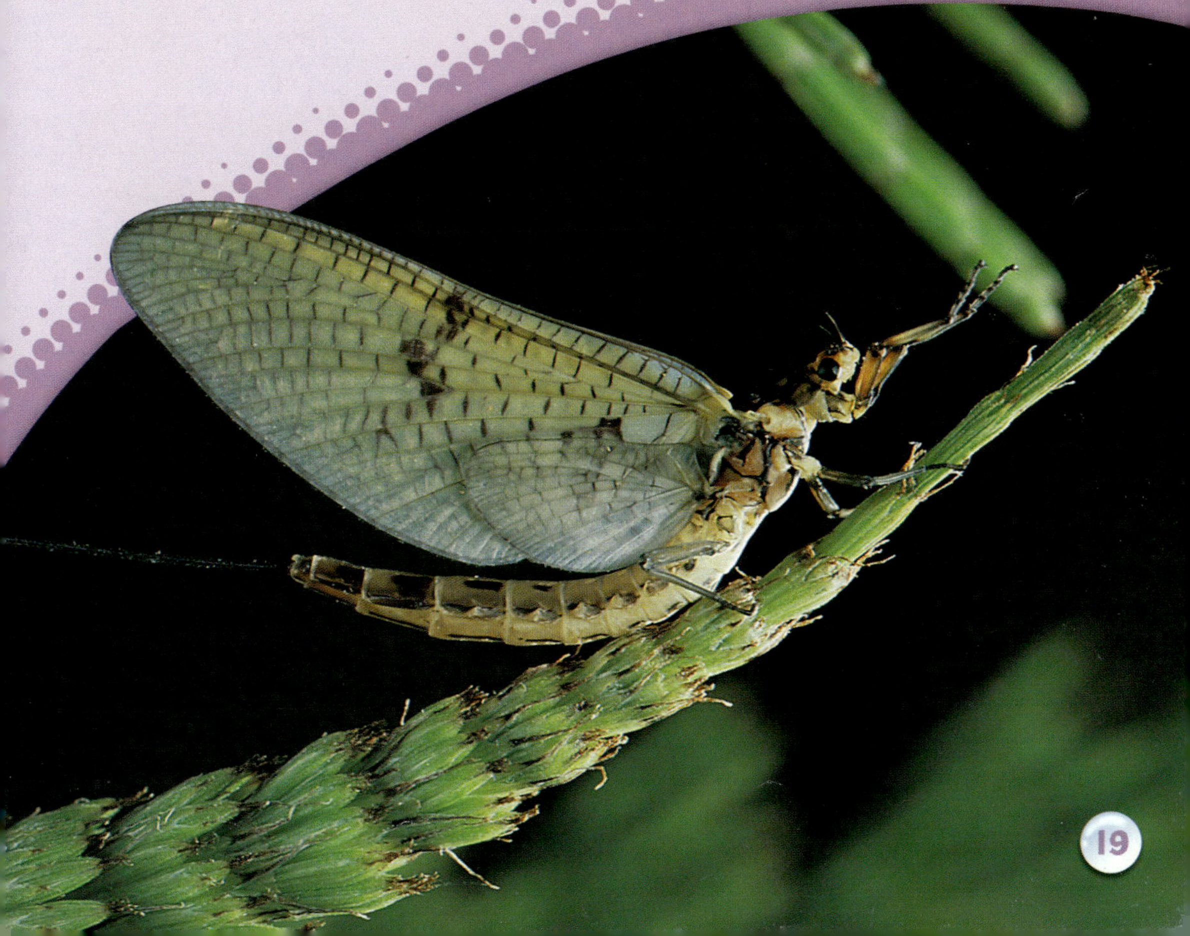

5 Minibeasts on You

Fleas and head lice visit people for a meal. They feed on blood. Your blood! First they prick your skin with their sharp mouths. Then they suck your blood!

? Did You Know?

A flea can jump more than 30 centimetres! That is the length of 100 fleas!

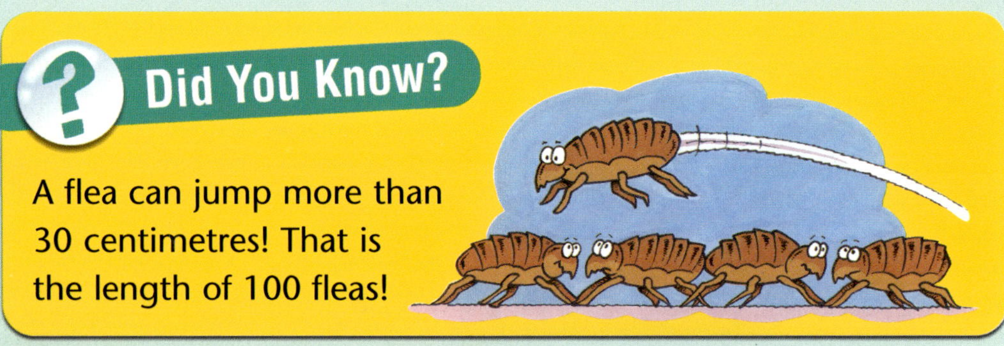

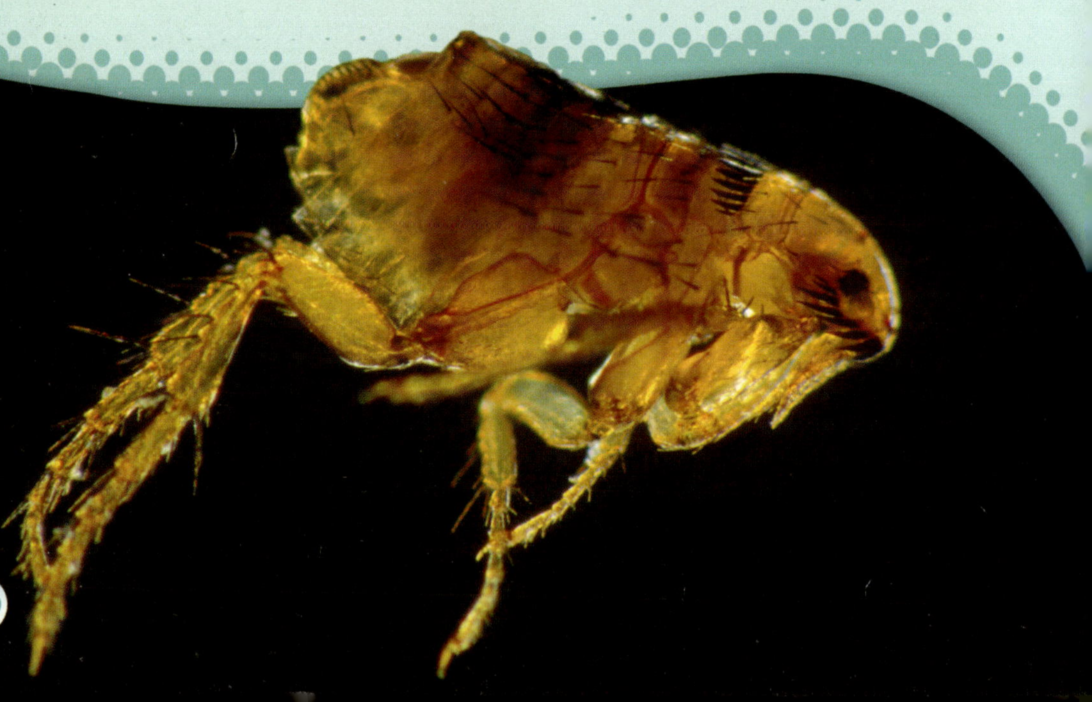

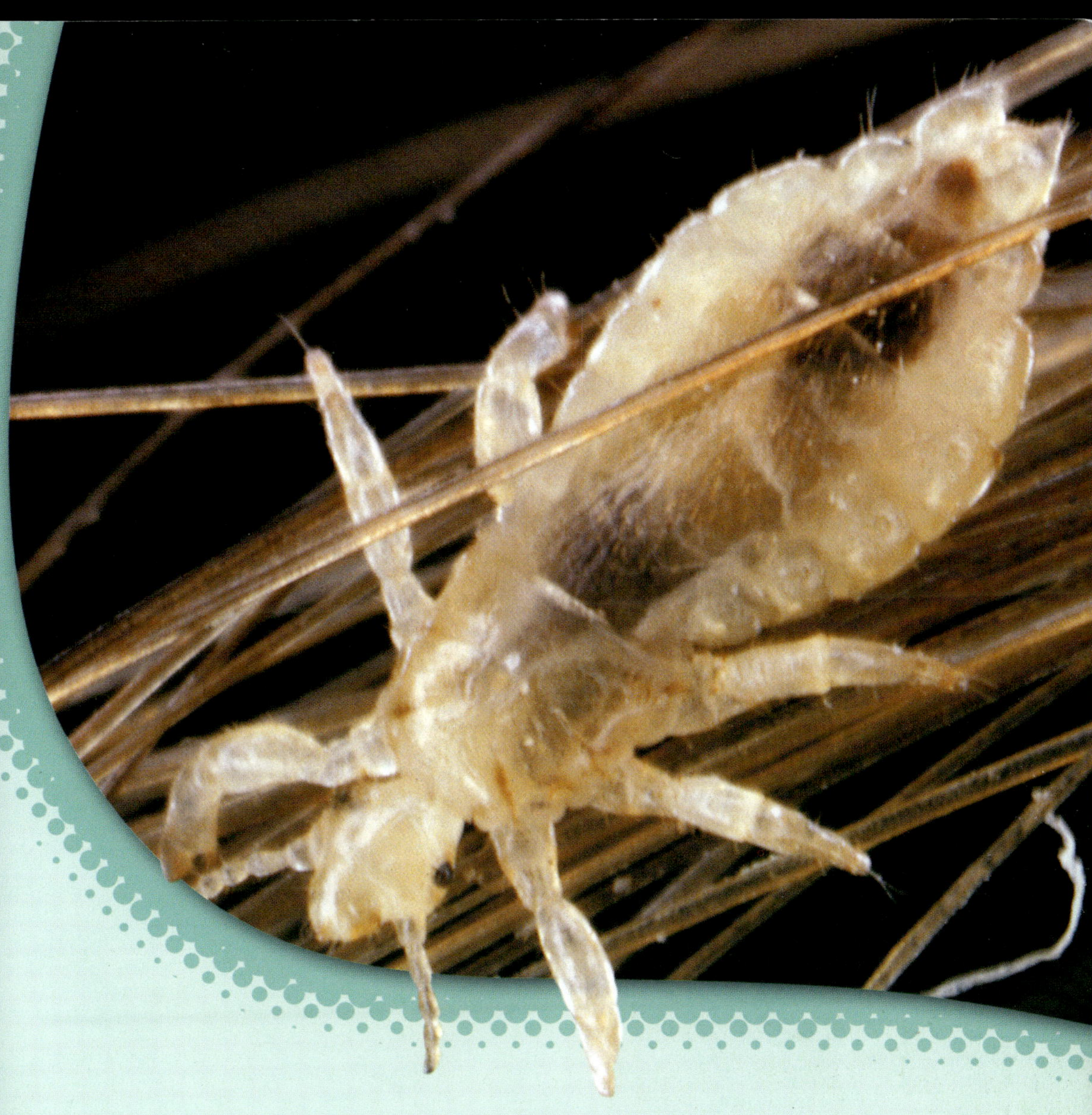

Head lice live in your hair – even if your hair is clean. Head lice cling to the hair on your head and lay eggs. They bite your head with their sharp mouth. Head lice suck blood every day.

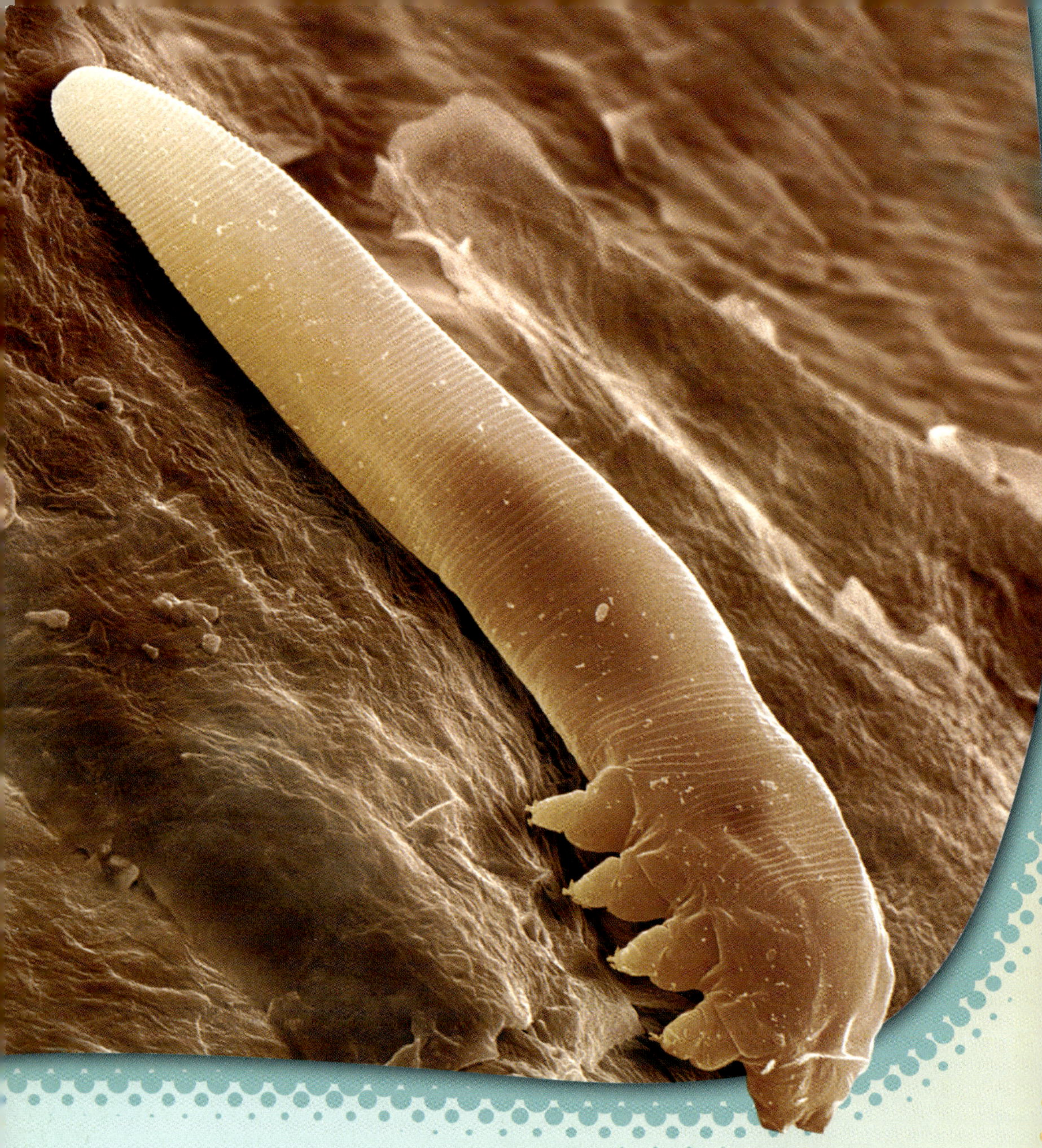

Tiny mites live on your eyelashes too. They eat bits of dead skin on your face. A female mite can lay up to 25 eggs on one eyelash!

6 Minibeasts Everywhere

Minibeasts live in the air, on land, in water and on you. They even live in books, but not new books like this one. Long ago, people stuck books together with glue. Some minibeasts eat this glue. They are called book lice!

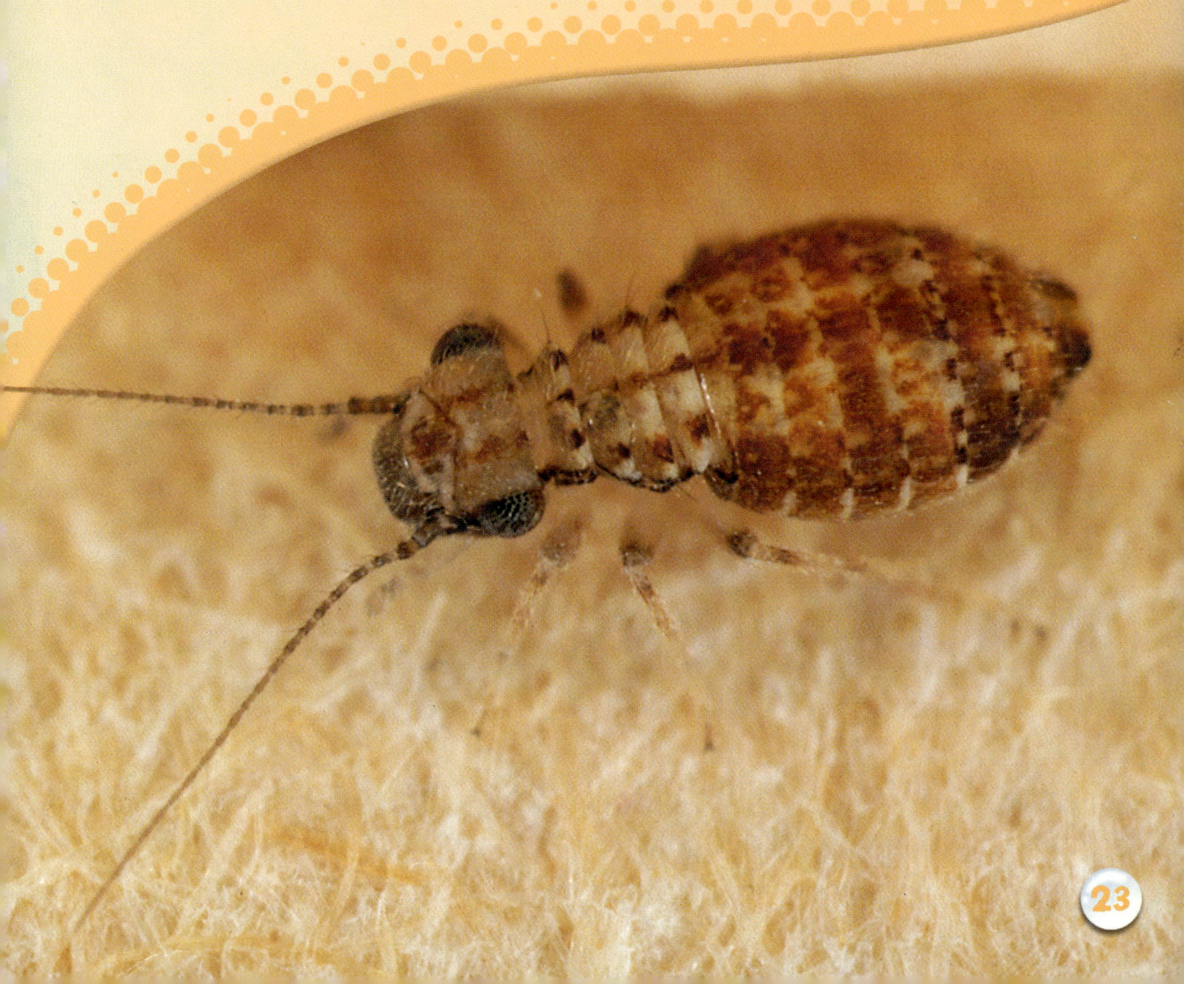

Index

Printed in Great Britain
by Amazon.co.uk, Ltd.,
Marston Gate.

This Is How You Recover From Depression

CONTENTS

PROLOGUE

When I graduated from high school in 2006, I was on top of the world. I'd been offered a scholarship to study Commerce/Law at Australia's most prestigious university, begun writing my first novel, had a great group of friends, and was going through a flattering phase of being approached by modelling scouts on the street on a monthly basis.

However, over the next couple of years, my world began to crumble, and I fell victim to a crippling depression. I grew sicker and sicker as the months wore on, and by April of 2010, my illness had suffocated the life out of me—as you can see from this excerpt from my memoir *Depression is a Liar*:

The days dragged along. This was the worst I'd ever felt. Period. There was no relief from the ceaseless dread. I could barely function. Paying attention in class was almost impossible. Studying was too overwhelming. I'd fallen absurdly behind. I hadn't touched my novel in days. I'd quit my part-time job at the law firm, too— needed all my free time to try and catch up on uni. But there was never enough time. I was constantly exhausted. Drained of life. Depression sucked at my soul. My spirit withered. My goal for the day got broken down even further: just survive the next six hours, I'd tell myself. The next four hours. Hold off killing yourself until then. [At which point, I'd tell myself the same thing over again].

I'd previously thought I'd get better. I'd always thought it true that hope and depression were bitter

rivals until one inevitably defeated the other, and I'd always thought that hope would win out in the end. But for the first time in my life, I was void of hope. I honestly believed that being depressed was just the way I was, and that being depressed was just the way I'd be, for the rest of my life. And because I was so convinced that I'd never get better, there seemed no point in fighting my illness. Instead of willing myself to "hang in there" because I believed that my suffering was temporary and that everything would be better one day, I comforted myself with the knowledge that human beings are not immortal. That I would die, one day. One special, glorious day. Then I could spend the rest of eternity moulding in a grave, free from pain. You might be wondering why I didn't just kill myself if I wholeheartedly believed that my future consisted of nothing more than excruciating misery. Well, first of all, I still was not a quitter. But more importantly, I didn't want to hurt the people that loved me.

It's not fair to commit suicide and ruin their lives, *I thought.* So I have to hold on. No matter how much it hurts me I have to hold on.

Hence why I drew comfort from the thought that one day I'd die and finally be free.

When you're that depressed, that insanely and utterly depressed that you genuinely believe you'll suffer that acutely for the rest of your days, life seems to lack all purpose.

After all, *I remember thinking,* what's the point in working, fighting, striving for a better life if I'm sentenced to one of chronic anguish and despair? There

is no better life. There is no life outside of pain. So what's the point in doing anything but waiting until death finally arrives on my doorstep and whisks me away to the Promised Land?

I was still studying, and I still planned on finishing my novel and trying to get it published, but it was more out of force of habit than anything else. My passion had been drained. My zest for life asphyxiated. I was like a ghost, just drifting through the ghastly days.

'Shit! What's wrong, mate?' an old friend once said when I ran into him at uni. 'Perk up, brother!'

I was shocked. One of the most well-known attributes of depression is that it is entirely possible—and very common—to suffer horrifically without anybody knowing. But somehow without realizing it, I'd crossed the line from a place where I was able to put on a front and fool people into thinking I wasn't depressed to a place where I was so sick that it was obvious to people I hadn't even seen for a year. When I got home I looked in the bathroom mirror, and realized that I was staring back at a man whose eyes were exhausted slits, whose whole face shrieked of agonizing misery. I was staring back at a man whose spirit had been broken, whose soul had been destroyed. I was staring back at a man who, for all intents and purposes, was already dead.

As you can see, I was so convinced I'd never get better. I was 100% sure of it. But over the next two years, I learned—with help from doctors, therapists, family members, friends and strangers alike—how to recover from my depression and find the happiness that had

been eluding me. My last episode was at the very beginning of 2012, and ever since then, I've been feeling great.

How this book will work

Recovering from depression and finding happiness again is one of the hardest things I've ever done, yet what I came to realise is that the process for doing so is relatively straightforward. In fact, I believe it can be broken down into three logical steps—and it's according to these three steps that this book will be structured.

Step 1: Understanding what is causing our depression

Depression is always caused by something—or a combination of things—and the first step in beating our illness is to understand exactly what's causing it.

In this part of the book, I'll tell you exactly what I did to work out what the causes of my depression were, and show you how you can do the same.

Step 2: Learning how to deal with the underlying causes of our depression so that they no longer depress us

In this section, we'll talk about how we can deal with some particularly common causes of depression, including spending too long doing things that we don't enjoy, loving ourselves for unhealthy reasons, holding onto anger, victimising ourselves, spending too much time with toxic people, being prisoners of what other people think of us, living an unbalanced life, perfectionism, living an unhealthy lifestyle, negative thinking, worrying about things that are out of our control, and several more.

Step 3: Learning how to handle a relapse

What I eventually learned is that if we're having a relapse, it means that right now, we're not yet able to manage the causes of our depression to an extent so masterful as to prevent them from depressing us. For this reason, if we experience a relapse, we need to go back and repeat steps one and two—i.e. we need to put more work into understanding what is causing that particular episode of depression, and then put more work into learning how to deal with

that cause so that it no longer has the power to trigger our depression.

If you repeat steps one and two every time you have a relapse, then like me, your relapses will gradually become less and less intense, and fewer and farther between. And in time, you can stop having relapses all together.

To quote a metaphor from *Depression is a Liar*:

> *It's as if there's a fortress surrounding our brains that's there to protect us from getting depressed, and every time we repeat steps one and two, another armed guard gets posted outside it. If depression's army still gets through from time to time, then it just means there aren't enough guards defending it yet. But if we keep repeating steps one and two, we will eventually have so many guards protecting us that depression's army will be shut out for good. It'll have no way of getting through.*

And it's because of this reason that if you follow this three step blueprint, then you really can recover from depression over time. It won't be easy, because you'll have to be proactive when you feel exhausted, you'll have to fight when you feel like giving up, and you'll have to remain hopeful when depression is doing everything in its power to break your will. But if you follow this three step process, you can get there in the end, because while it's hard for a person to beat depression, it's even harder for depression to beat a person who never gives up.

Step 1:
Understanding what is causing our depression

CHAPTER 1

"You cannot overcome what you refuse to confront."

As you may already know, clinical depression can be caused by one or more of the following things:

- A chemical imbalance in our brains;
- Our behaviours (for example, spending time with toxic people);
- Our circumstances (for example, doing a job we don't enjoy);
- Our thought processes (for example, concluding that we're unattractive and unlovable if someone says "no" to going on a date with us);
- Life events (for example, going through a messy break-up).

And, like we've said, in order to recover from depression, we need to figure out precisely what's causing it. Trying to recover without taking the time to do so is analogous to trying to stop a ship from sinking when we've got no idea where the water's getting in from. Try all we want, but we're going to keep sinking.

To help us understand what might be causing our depression, we can do the following.

See a psychiatrist (or a good GP)

Like we've said, depression can sometimes be caused by a chemical imbalance in our brains. In the case of unipolar depression, this is due to a lack of serotonin, dopamine, adrenalin or noradrenalin. Alternatively, depression can often be part of another illness that involves a different sort of chemical imbalance, such as bipolar disorder (depression coupled with mania). Either way, one of the most important things to do if we suffer from depression is to see a psychiatrist (or if that isn't feasible, a good GP). Their job is to correctly diagnose us, and if they then deem it appropriate, to prescribe us medication to manage our chemical imbalance.

Seeing a psychiatrist and taking medication was crucial to my recovery. For the record, I was diagnosed with bipolar disorder at the end of 2010, and medication helped keep me on the straight and narrow until November of 2014, when my psychiatrist said I no longer needed to take it.

See a therapist

The reason why it's so important to see a therapist is because part of their role is to determine the behaviours, circumstances, thought processes and life events that may be causing our depression.

Seeing a therapist is crucial to recovering from depression, but a lot of people don't

see one—often because they think that seeing a doctor and taking medication will be enough. But as we've intimated, the role of a doctor and a therapist are *not* the same. Again, a doctor's role is to accurately diagnose us, and if necessary, to prescribe us medication to balance the chemicals in our brains; on the other hand, a therapist's job is to analyse our behaviours, circumstances, thought processes and the events that have taken place in our lives to work out what may be causing our depression, and then to teach us how to deal with these underlying causes. *So if we see one but not the other, we're missing out on some vital treatment that is crucial to our recovery.*

Start keeping a mood diary

Before you go to bed every night, take note of what you did that day, and rank how you felt that day out of 10—with 10 being very happy, and one being suicidally depressed. For example:

Activity	Time
Sleeping	12:00am – 8:00am
Having a shower	8:00am-8:15am
Having breakfast with my wife	8:15am-8:45am
Travelling to work while listening to music	8:45am-9:30am
Working by myself at my desk	9:30am-11:30am
Having coffee with my friend Bob	11:30am-12:15pm
Work meeting with Jeff and Susie	12:15pm-1:30pm
Having lunch in the sun with my friend Jane	1:30pm-2:15pm
Work meeting with Phil	2:15pm-3:15pm
Working by myself at my desk	3:15pm-4:15pm
Work meeting with Brad, Peter and Ron	4:15pm-4:45pm
Working by myself at my desk	4:45pm-6:00pm
Travelling home reading a book	6:00pm-6:45pm
Going for a run	6:45pm-7:45pm
Eating dinner with my family	7:45pm-9:00pm
Watching television with my wife	9:00pm-10:00pm
Listening to music to try and relax	10:00pm-11:15pm
Getting ready for bed/work the next day	11:15pm-12:00am
How I felt today	**8/10**

After a while, you'll notice that days when you feel depressed correlate to you doing certain activities—or not doing certain activities—and this can help you work out what may be causing your depression.

For example, when I used to keep mood diaries, it helped me work out that drinking alcohol really triggered my depression. Over time, I noticed that if I went out on a Saturday evening for a big night, I'd often find myself feeling down on Tuesday, Wednesday or Thursday. After noticing this trend, I decided to significantly reduce how much alcohol I drank on weekends, and low and behold, I began noticing an upward trend in my mood on Tuesdays, Wednesdays and Thursdays. I thus concluded that drinking too much alcohol contributed to me feeling depressed—something I may not have worked out if I hadn't kept a mood diary.

In terms of how to logistically keep a mood diary, I recommend using a regular diary to record what you're doing each day, and Mood Tracker to document your mood. This tool's graphical feature shows your daily mood level, as well as how many hours you slept that night and what dosage of medication you're taking (if any). In addition to being a handy mood tracking tool, it also has a public forum where you can share your mood chart and medication records with other people going through similar things as you. Moreover, you can schedule text messages or emails to be periodically sent to you to remind you to take your medication.

Talk to someone we're close with about what they think makes us depressed

If we spend a lot of time with someone, then sometimes they will notice a lot about our mood that we don't always pick up on, and these insights can be really valuable in helping us understand what's causing our depression. For example, our partner may notice that when we don't get a good night's sleep, we're really cranky and crabby the next day. Similarly, our kids might notice that we're tense and irritable if we don't exercise for a week.

Key takeaways from this chapter

In order to determine what's causing our depression, we want to:

1/ See a doctor (preferably a psychiatrist);

2/ See a therapist;

3/ Keep a mood diary;

4/ Talk to someone we're close with about what *they* think makes *us* depressed.

Each of these things is worth doing. If we only do one or two of them, then we're likely to miss out on identifying a couple of the things that cause us to feel depressed. This is really going to slow down our recovery, and if it's a particularly key cause, the reality is that it's likely to keep us trapped in depression forever.

Step 2: Learning how to deal with the underlying causes of our depression so that they no longer depress us

CHAPTER 2
Common Cause of People's Depression #1:
Spending too long doing things that we don't enjoy doing

"Happiness is not something readymade—it comes from your own actions."
Dalai Lama

Have you ever watched the movie *Dead Poets Society*? If not, I'd highly recommend it, because its plot can give you powerful insight into the human psyche, and the kind of things that can trigger your depression.

The main character, Neil Perry, wants to be an actor, but he knows his father will disapprove. Without telling him, he auditions for the role of Puck in Shakespeare's *A Midsummer Night's Dream*, and he gets it. To cut a long story short, his father finds out, and demands that Neil withdraw from the play. When Neil doesn't, he tells his son that he is going to enrol him in a military school, after which Neil would go to Harvard to study medicine. Unable to face such a prospect, Neil then gets his grandfather's gun, and kills himself.

A tragic story, no doubt, and one that raises a very, very important point: a big trigger for a lot of people—including myself when I used to suffer from depression—is spending lots of time doing things that don't make us happy, and very little time doing things that do make us happy.

During my interaction with thousands of people who suffer from depression, I've noticed that this generally occurs for four main reasons:

1/ Many of us just don't know what makes us happy and what doesn't make us happy;

2/ Even if we do know what makes us happy and what doesn't make us happy, many of us aren't good at structuring our lives in such a way that we maximise the time we spend doing things that make us happy and minimise the time we spend doing things that don't make us happy;

3/ Like our friend in *Dead Poets Society*, many of us don't do what we enjoy doing because of pressure from others to do something else;

4/ Sometimes our inflexible circumstances make it difficult for us to do a lot of what makes us happy.

Let's now deal with each of these four issues in turn.

What makes us happy?

In order to figure out what makes us happy, there are a number of things that we can do.

Set aside some time to identify our core values

When I say "identify our core values", what I mean is identifying those things that mean the most to us in the world.

Ask yourself, *what gets me excited?*

What inspires me?

What gives me a buzz?

What am I thinking about during those times when I'm lying in bed and I feel so alive that I can't fall asleep? (I know if you're suffering from depression then this may be difficult to remember, but really try. Really try to think about what gets you going).

Is it helping people?

Is it making money?

Is it spending time with your friends and family?

Is it being artistic—like playing a musical instrument, singing or writing a book?

Is it travelling?

Is it sport?

I could go on and on, but what I'm saying is that we all need to be in touch with our core values, because once we're in touch with them, we can then go about restructuring our lives so that we spend as much time as possible doing things that satisfy our core values. And it's when we're doing this that we'll be our happiest selves.

For example, two of my primary core values are being creative (by writing books) and helping people. However, when I was at university I studied Commerce/Law—a degree which would've led to a career in law, investment banking, or management consulting. Those sorts of careers are much more congruent with satisfying a core value along the lines of "making lots of money", as opposed to satisfying the core values of being creative or helping people. As a result, I was miserable studying Commerce/Law, and the mere idea of going into that line of work would make me feel suicidal—much like a career in medicine did for Neil Perry in *Dead Poets Society*. Now, I'm certainly not knocking being a lawyer, an investment banker or a management consultant—they're great jobs if they satisfy *your* core values. But, they didn't satisfy *my* core values, and as a result, pursuing such a career didn't make me happy. For no other reason, I eventually quit my Commerce/Law degree at the start of 2012, and as soon as I did, and as soon as I started focusing on

satisfying my core values of being creative and helping people, I started feeling much, much happier. In fact, I haven't had a depressive episode ever since.

Talk to someone we're close with about what they think makes us happy

The second thing we can do to try and work out what makes us happy is to talk to someone we're close with about what *they* think makes *us* happy.

For example, my brother loves food. I mean, he *really* loves food. If we go out for a really tasty breakfast in the morning, he'll be on a high all day—seriously, he'll be significantly more elevated, inspired and vibrant after he's had a nice meal. After we'd been backpacking around Asia for a couple of months together, I started to pick up on this trend, and I asked him:

'Mat, do you notice that whenever you eat a meal you really enjoy, you're so much more lively for the rest of the day?'

'No,' he replied, 'I'd never noticed that before. But you're right––I *am* always in a particularly good mood after I eat a nice meal'.

This insight helped my brother better understand what makes him happy, and from that moment on, he's been able to use this information to make decisions that have led him to be happier. For example, he now makes a thoughtful effort to eat an enjoyable meal whenever he can afford it—as opposed to wasting his money on something else that doesn't impact him in as positive a way.

Expose ourselves to new activities

The third thing we can do to try and work out what makes us happy is to expose ourselves to new activities with the hopes of finding a new hobby and to meet new groups of people. Here are some tips to help us do so:

1/ **When considering a new hobby, we need to think about what's feasible for our lifestyle and budget.** For example, if we live 500 kilometres inland, then surfing isn't a suitable hobby—but keeping a garden might be.

2/ **Go back to our core values.** Whether it's making money, spending time with loved ones or doing something creative, thinking about the things that mean the most to us can help us identify potential new hobbies.

3/ **Go back in time.** Most of us have things that we loved doing when we were younger, but then at some point life got in the way and we stopped doing them. If we're looking for new hobbies now, however, then it's a good time to revisit those things.

4/ **Join a friend.** Next time one of our friends is going somewhere to pursue one of their hobbies, we can tag along with them.

To give you a few ideas to think about, I've put together the following list of potential hobbies, organised into various categories. It's by no means exhaustive, but it should serve as a starting point to get your mind ticking:

- **Something creative:** writing, painting, drawing, singing, dancing, playing a musical instrument, sculpting, pottery, origami, calligraphy, scrap-booking or jewellery making.

- **Something intellectual:** reading, learning another language, philosophy, history, taking an open university course or studying part-time.
- **Something active:** playing a sport, running, going to the gym, swimming, rock climbing, cycling, skiing, snowboarding, bodybuilding or martial arts.
- **Something extreme:** skydiving, bungee jumping, base jumping, motor cycling, hangliding or white water rafting.
- **Something outdoors:** kite flying, camping, snorkelling, scuba diving, gardening, fishing, bush walking, caving, bird watching, star gazing, hiking, paintball, photography, sailing, noodling, restoring old cars, horse riding, canoeing or kite surfing.
- **Something spiritual:** yoga or meditation.
- **Something social:** hanging out with friends, listening to live music, going to the movies, going to trivia nights, getting involved in local events, or wine tasting.
- **Something indoors:** puzzles, card games, board games, dominoes, video games, museums, art galleries, darts, billiards, fantasy sports or woodwork.
- **Something financial:** investing, share trading or building financial models.
- **Volunteer work:** founding a charity about a cause you care about, doing volunteer work for an existing charity, organising a fundraiser or coaching a local sports team.
- **Start a collection:** of stamps, postcards, antiques, trading cards, coins, rocks or minerals.
- **Travelling.**
- **Get a pet.**

Keep a mood diary

The fourth thing we can do to try and work out what makes us happy is to keep a mood diary. This is a concept that we talked about earlier on in the context of trying to figure out what's triggering our depression, but keeping a mood diary is also an invaluable exercise that can help us figure out what makes us happy.

To refresh your memory about how a mood diary works, before you go to sleep every night, write down everything you did that day, and rank your mood out of 10—10 being very happy, and one being miserably suicidal. After a while, you'll notice that days when you're in a good mood correlate to you having done—or not having done—certain activities, and days when you're depressed correlate to you having done—or not having done—other activities.

For example, one of the things I identified from keeping a mood diary was that days I spent in the sun were days when I was in a better mood. When I noticed this, I raised it with my psychologist.

'That's not surprising,' he said. 'We get Vitamin D from the sun, and Vitamin D increases our serotonin levels.'

Ever since making this observation, I've thus made a deliberate effort to do most of my writing outdoors, and I'm in a really great mood whenever I do so. This is another example of how knowing what makes us happy allows us to then take deliberate actions that will lead us to be happy.

On the other hand, however, if we don't know what makes us happy, then it's really difficult to make the decisions that we need to make or to take the actions that we need to take in order for us to be

happy. Or, put another way, it's really *easy* for us to make decisions and take actions that will lead us to be *unhappy*—or even worse, that will lead us to be depressed.

Let technology help us!

The great thing about living in the 21st century is that there are apps and tools (most of which are free) that can help us do plenty of the things that we want to do—including determining what makes us happy. One app I'd particularly recommend is the Happy Habits app. This app features a 119 question quiz covering 14 factors that affect your mood, and based on your answers, Happy Habits will provide suggestions to create more happiness in your life. The app also includes a "happiness journal" for you to record affirmations and positive events, in addition to articles about cognitive behavioural therapy and happiness.

Another really helpful app is Secret of Happiness. Every morning for 30 days, the app asks you to think of a reason to be happy, and every night, it asks you to think about something you did that day that made you happy. The creators of the app believe that by training your mind in this way to be more aware of what makes you happy, you may find that at the end of 30 days, you know the secrets to your happiness.

How to structure our lives in such a way as to maximise our happiness

If we take the time to identify our core values, talk to people close to us about what *they* think makes *us* happy, expose ourselves to knew activities, keep a mood diary, and use a cleverly developed happiness app or two, then after a while, we're going to really understand what makes us happy. However, this knowledge is next to useless if we don't then use it to structure our lives in such a way that we maximise the time we spend doing things that make us happy, and minimise the time we spend doing things that don't make us happy.

I've noticed that the main reason we often struggle with this implementation process is because we can be prone to putting up roadblocks that stop us from actually making the changes that we need to make in order to be happier.

Let's talk about some of those roadblocks now.

Saying we don't have time

Let's be perfectly honest with ourselves: what we *really* mean when we say that we "don't have time" to do something is that we're choosing not to make that something a priority. Let's look at a really common example of going to the gym. Literally speaking, we *all* have time to go to the gym—there are 24 hours in a day, and going to the gym takes around an hour. Yes, we have a bunch of other things that we need to do in those 24 hours too, but that's my point——when we say that we "don't have time" to go to the gym one day,

what we're really saying is that for that 24 hour period, we're prioritising doing 24 hours' worth of other things over going to the gym.

The reason I make this point is that in order to recover from depression—and in order to be happy in general—we can't afford *not* to prioritise doing things that make us happy. Put another way, in order to be our happiest selves, we need to make sure that we are allocating as many of our 24 hours as possible to activities we enjoy.

In my experience, the easiest way to prioritise the things that make us happy is to set aside a dedicated block of time for them in our schedule. Then, all we have to do is stick to our timetable. I do this with reading, for example. It's something I absolutely love to do, but I find that it's one of those things where, if I don't set aside blocks of time to do it, then other things come up and it often falls by the wayside. For this reason, I set aside an hour every morning to read, and that's how I make sure I find time to do it.

In order to help you prioritise your time, I recommend using the Way of Life app. Marketed as the "ultimate habit maker and breaker", this app helps you set goals and then track whether or not you're achieving them on a daily or weekly basis. Alternatively, you might like to use the Daily Routine app, which is designed to keep busy people on task. This app will keep track of your schedule and send you notifications about what you should be doing and when. You can schedule routines for specific days of the week or month, and have special reminders sent to you for tasks you're worried you might forget. The app also syncs with your online calendar, to include new events as they are scheduled.

Fear of change is another thing that can be an impediment to us restructuring our lives so that we're doing more of what makes us happy and less of what doesn't make us happy. For example, I used to study Commerce/Law as you know, and as a result, I know a lot of people who followed the path of becoming lawyers or investment bankers or management consultants. Unfortunately, I also know for a fact that a lot of them hate their jobs. They've told me things like, 'instead of being a lawyer, I wish I was a journalist'; or 'I wish I could teach scuba diving instead of being a management consultant'.

'Mate, you could still be a journalist,' I've said to them before 'You're only 24! You still have the opportunity to do pretty much anything you want to!'

'No, I don't,' they'd reply. 'I've spent close to a decade working my ass off to become a lawyer. I can't give up on that now.'

I can relate to that line of thinking, because it held me back for a long time as well.

I've spent five or six years building up my career, I remember thinking. *I've studied so hard and put so much effort into padding my resume with work experience and other extracurricular activities to get one of those top corporate jobs . . . am I really going to throw all of that away now? And particularly since I'm getting so close to graduating?*

The prospect of giving up everything I'd worked so hard for was terrifying, but what scared me even more was knowing that if I continued along the path I was on—that of becoming a lawyer or an investment banker or a management consultant and completely ignoring my core values of being creative and helping people—then I would never be happy. So I made a huge career change, and I've never regretted it since.

If you're in a similar position with respect to your career, your relationship, or in another area of your life, then I encourage you to think about taking a similar sort of leap. I know change can be scary as hell, but ask yourself: is it scarier than the prospect of being unhappy for the rest of your life?

Wasting time on things that don't make us happy

A few months ago on my Facebook fan page, I asked everyone:

What do you think is the biggest impediment to making you happy?

To my surprise, one of the most common responses was "wasting time" on things that at the end of the day, "don't contribute much to making us happy". This included, to quote the responses, "spending time on Facebook", "watching the news or mediocre television shows", "browsing the internet", or "reading trashy magazines".

If we find ourselves in this position, then we need to remind ourselves of all the things we have in our lives that do make us happy, and make a determined effort to do those things. Like we've said, scheduling those activities into our days is a good way to make sure that we'll have time to do them, and if it's distracting websites that's causing us to waste time, then a solution we haven't mentioned yet it using the SelfControl app. This app lets you block access to websites of your choice for a pre-defined period of time, thereby forcing you to focus on something else.

Pressure from other people

The scenario in *Dead Poets Society* is not an uncommon one, and it doesn't just happen in the parent/child context. For example, often it's our partners that pressure us to enter or stay in a career that we really don't like, just because it's more financially attractive than the one we'd prefer.

This is a really tough situation to be in, and I don't think there's an easy way out of it. In my opinion, if we find ourselves in such a position, then the first step we should take is to sit down with the person who's pressuring us and try to explain to them that we don't like what we're doing and that we'd much rather do something else. It's best to be really open, honest and genuine here, because I've found that if we are, then there's a good chance that the person will understand, and stop pressuring us into living a life we don't want. After all, our loved ones don't like to see us suffering, do they?

However, there are times when the other person just won't budge. I've heard people say to their children and partner things like "until you retire, you don't have time to be happy—you have to build your career and make as much money as possible"; and, I've had people look at me like I was from outer space when I told them that I was going to quit Commerce/Law to pursue my dream of becoming an author. People who think like this will in all likelihood never understand us if we tell them that we want to pursue a different path in the name of happiness. And when we're dealing with these people, we have a couple of choices.

Firstly, we could give in to their pressure and just keep doing what we're doing. Sometimes circumstances dictate that we have to do this—such as if we need to keep our high-paying-but-uninspiring job because we have a mortgage to pay off (see next section).

However, I wouldn't recommend doing this if it is possible not to. If we find ourselves in such a position, there's a reason why treading the path we're on is making us miserable, and that's because it's not the right one for us. Continuing to stumble down it might preserve our relationship with those people who are pressuring us to do so, but it will just make us more and more unhappy.

Alternatively, we could begin to distance ourselves from these people—which is the option that I personally took and the one I'd recommend insofar as it is possible. The way I saw it, anyone who valued my happiness so minimally that they'd rather see me be miserable than pursue something I enjoy is not someone I consider a good influence on my life. And secondly, anyone who would rather me pursue something I hate as opposed to something I enjoy has an entirely different set of values to me—in the dropping-out-of-Commerce/Law scenario, this was the prioritising of money over more or less everything else—and, as we'll talk about later on, we're unlikely to have happy, healthy relationships with people who have vastly different values to us anyway.

What if our inflexible circumstances make it difficult to do what makes us happy?

Like we just alluded to, there are times when we may be forced to continue doing something that we don't particularly enjoy because of less than flexible circumstances—the most common example being sticking with an unenjoyable but well-paying job to pay off the mortgage or the school fees. While we may not be able to change

our job in such a scenario, there are a number of things we can do to make it more bearable.

1/ **Remind ourselves of the reasons why we're doing it.** Ask yourself, *what's the reason I'm making this sacrifice?* Then, remind yourself of it every single day. Focusing on the fruits of our labour can make the labour itself a whole lot more tolerable.

2/ **Make sure we enjoy the fruits of our labour.** For example, if the reason we're working an unenjoyable but high-paying job is to put our kids through a private school, then we can make a point of getting involved in our children's school activities. Doing this helps us focus on the reason why we're making the sacrifice that we're making, which like we've said, can make our job itself more endurable.

3/ **In our *free* time, make a point of maximising the time we spend on enjoyable activities and minimising the time we spend doing unenjoyable activities.** Like we've said, this is something that everybody ought to do, but it's even more important if we're forced to do a job we don't particularly like. In such a case, if we're at least spending our leisure time doing things we find pleasurable, then it can help sustain us during our working hours.

4/ **Make our unenjoyable job as enjoyable as can be.** We might not be able to quit our job, but in many cases, there are things we can do to make it more enjoyable. For example, getting involved in inter-office social activities, changing projects, or changing departments.

Key takeaways from this chapter

1/ If we can structure our lives in such a way that we maximise the time we spend doing things that make us happy and minimise the time we spend doing things that don't make us happy, then we will take gigantic strides towards recovering from depression and returning to living the life we want.

2/ We can understand more about what makes us happy by:

a) Identifying our core values;
b) Talking to people we're close with about what they think makes us happy;
c) Exposing ourselves to new activities;
d) Keeping a mood diary;
e) Using nifty apps and tools like Happy Habits or Secret of Happiness.

3/ There are five common obstacles that often prevent us from implementing the changes that we need to make in our lives in order to maximise the time we spend doing the things that make us happy and minimise the time we spend doing the things that don't make us happy. These include:

a) Saying we don't have time;
b) Fear;
c) Wasting time on things that don't add to our happiness;
d) Pressure from other people;
e) Inflexible circumstances.

4/ We can do the following to help us overcome such obstacles:

a) Schedule time to do the things that make us happy, and be disciplined about following that schedule.

b) Acknowledge that while change can be scary, continuing down a path that we know is making us miserable is pretty damn scary too, and that for this reason, perhaps change is actually the lesser of two fears.

c) Have an honest, open-hearted talk with the person who is pressuring us to do something that we really don't like doing. If they listen and understand, they're likely to ease up on us; however, if they don't listen or understand, then we may want to consider distancing ourselves from that person.

d) If we're somewhat shackled by inflexible circumstances, we can make the best of our situation by reminding ourselves of the reasons why we're making the sacrifices we're making, by ensuring that we enjoy the fruits of our labour, by making sure we do what we enjoy in our leisure time, and by making our unenjoyable job as enjoyable as can be.

CHAPTER 3
Common Cause of People's Depression #2:
Loving ourselves for unhealthy reasons, or not loving ourselves at all

"I have an everyday religion that works for me. Love yourself first, and everything else falls into line."
Lucille Ball

Many of us who suffer from depression do not love ourselves. Or, even if we do love ourselves, it's entirely possible that the love we have for ourselves is based on a foundation that's relatively unstable; this in turn means that *we* will be relatively unstable, which makes us an easy target for Depression (and he's a hell of a good shooter). If you've read my memoir *Depression is a Liar*, you'll know that loving myself for unhealthy reasons was one of the biggest, if not *the* biggest cause of my depression. Learning how to love myself for healthy reasons was thus crucial to my recovery, and for this reason, this particular chapter is one that's very close to my heart.

We'll start by talking about some of the really "healthy" reasons why we can love ourselves. Then, we'll go on to talk about some of the really "unhealthy" reasons why people love themselves, and demonstrate how basing our love for ourselves on one or all of these reasons can lead us to become extremely unstable—and thus extremely depressed.

Healthy reasons to love ourselves

Healthy reasons to love ourselves can be divided into two categories:

1/ Our skills—i.e. things that we're good at;

2/ Our personal qualities and characteristics.

These "reasons to love ourselves" are healthy because they are:

1/ In our control;

2/ Independent of what other people think of us;

3/ Independent of circumstances.

As I've said, loving myself for healthy reasons is something I really used to struggle with, but over the years, it's a skill I've worked very hard to master. In the course of doing so, I once wrote down the following list of healthy reasons to love myself, which I used to read through all the time so that they'd become ingrained in my mind.

- *I love myself because I'm a kind person—someone who always tries to treat other people with respect.*
- *I love myself because I'm an honest person who acts with integrity.*
- *I love myself because I have the determination and the work ethic to pursue my dreams through to completion.*
- *I love myself because I have the courage to face my problems and deal with them, instead of denying that they exist.*
- *I love myself because I'm a compassionate person who helps other people.*
- *I love myself because I'm intelligent.*
- *I love myself because I'm a good writer.*
- *I love myself because I'm a fighter—because I had the strength to turn my life around and transform myself from*

the extremely suicidal person I was into the extremely happy person that I am today.

These are all healthy reasons to love myself, and because my love for myself is based upon reasons that are healthy—i.e. reasons that are in my control, independent of circumstances, and independent of what other people think of me—I am an emotionally stable person, which contributes to me being very happy.

How does loving ourselves for healthy reasons lead us to be emotionally stable?

Let's say that, for example, a girl I ask on a date turns me down. In such an instance, I would feel disappointed, of course. However, because I love myself for healthy reasons, I wouldn't then conclude that I'm "unattractive", "ugly", "unlovable" or anything else of the sort, nor would I go to pieces and spiral into depression. On the contrary, my self-esteem would remain high, and I'd still feel emotionally stable.

Why?

Because a girl turning me down for a date has no impact on the reasons why I love myself.

Let's return to my list.

I love myself because I'm a kind person—someone who always tries to treat other people with respect.

Does a girl turning me down for a date mean that I'm no longer a kind person? Or that I no longer treat other people with respect? No, it doesn't mean that at all.

Next reason: *I love myself because I'm an honest person who acts with integrity.*

Does the fact that a girl turned me down for a date mean that that's no longer true? Of course not.

Third reason: *I love myself because I have the determination and the work ethic to pursue my dreams through to completion.*

Once again, a girl turning me down for a date has no impact on this reason why I love myself. After all, despite being turned down, I am still a determined person who works hard.

Fourth reason: *I love myself because I have the courage to face my problems and deal with them, instead of denying that they exist.*

Once again, does a girl turning me down for a date change that? Does it mean that I no longer have the courage to face my problems and deal with them instead of denying that they exist? Not at all.

I can go through this analysis for each of the reasons on my list and arrive at the same conclusion every time—because as we've said, each of the reasons on my list are *healthy* reasons to love myself. For this reason, if a girl turns me down for a date, instead of falling apart, I can instead think:

OK, a girl turned me down . . . that's disappointing, but at the same time, I still know I'm a good person. I know I still have a lot to offer a girl. And, even though this particular girl didn't want to get to know me better, I know there's another one out there who will.

Let me give you another example. Let's say that someone disagrees with an article I write about depression, and they decide to send me an email saying that it's terrible and that I'm an idiot and that I have no idea what I'm talking about. If this happened, I wouldn't exactly be jumping up and down, but at the same time, it's not going to shatter my self-esteem or cause me to go to pieces. In

reality, it's going to have very little effect on me. Why? Because once again, it has no impact on the reasons why I love myself—and because it has no impact on the reasons why I love myself, I still love myself just as much as I did before that person sent me an abusive email.

The running theme is this: I love myself for reasons that I am in control of, that are independent of what other people think of me, and that are independent of circumstances. For this reason, no-one can take them away from me—not a girl, not someone who disagrees with something I write, not anyone. I don't need them—or anyone else—to validate my own love for myself. And this is critically important, because it means that when something goes wrong or when I'm facing adversity, my self-esteem remains high, and I don't go to pieces.

What happens if our love for ourselves is based on unhealthy reasons?

Now let's talk about what happens if our love for ourselves is based on what I like to call "unhealthy" reasons. For example:

1/ If we were to love ourselves because our partner loves us;

2/ If we were to love ourselves because our boss likes the job we do at work;

3/ If we were to love ourselves because our business is going well.

Now you may ask: *why are these "unhealthy" reasons to love ourselves?*

And my answer is this: the reason that these reasons to love ourselves are unhealthy is because they are *not* in our control, they are *not* independent of circumstances, and they are *not* independent of what other people think of us. This is very dangerous, because it leaves us extremely vulnerable to falling victim to depression—as we can see in each of the following examples.

If one of the fundamental reasons why we love ourselves is because our partner loves us, then imagine how we're going to feel if that person breaks up with us. Firstly, just like someone who loves themselves for healthy reasons will be, we're going to be heartbroken. However, *unlike* someone who loves themselves for healthy reasons, we're also likely to think all sorts of thoughts like:

Wow, my partner broke up with me . . . that must mean that I'm unlovable . . . and if I'm unlovable, then that must mean that no-one will ever love me again . . . and if no-one will ever love me again,

then that must mean that I'll never find another partner . . . and if I never find another partner, then that means I'm going to spend the rest of my life miserable and alone.

If we love ourselves because our partner loves us, then we're likely to catastrophize the break-up like so, which is going to destroy our self-esteem and plunge us into an awful spell of depression.

Let's take another example: we love ourselves because our boss likes the work we do, but then we get a new boss who doesn't particularly appreciate our input. If this happens, then just like someone who loves themselves for healthy reasons will be, we're going to feel disappointed. However, *unlike* someone who loves themselves for healthy reasons, we're also likely to catastrophize the situation and think all kinds of poisonous thoughts like:

Oh, my new boss doesn't appreciate my work . . . that must mean I'm a terrible worker . . . and because I'm a terrible worker, I'm probably going to get fired soon . . . and because I'm a terrible worker, I'll probably never be able to get another job once I get fired . . . so I'm probably going to be unemployed for years on end.

Once again, catastrophizing this issue like so is going to cripple our self-esteem and trigger our depression.

Last example: we love ourselves because our business is doing well, but then the economy crashes and our business goes with it. Again, just like someone who loves themselves for healthy reasons, we're going to feel absolutely shattered. However, *unlike* someone who loves themselves for healthy reasons, we're also likely to catastrophize the situation and think things like:

My business crashed because I'm an idiot . . . and because I'm an idiot, I'll never be able to start another business again . . . and because I'll never be able to start another business again, I'll always be broke . . . and because I'll always be broke, I'll always be miserable . . . and because I'll always be broke and miserable, I'll never be able to attract a partner . . . which means I'll never be able

to have a family . . . which means I'm going to die broke, miserable, and all alone.

The running theme is this: when we base our love for ourselves on what other people think of us or on circumstances that are out of our control, we give those people and those circumstances so much power over our own happiness. And because we can't control those people or those circumstances—they can change at any minute—it means that when adversity strikes us, we're going to catastrophize everything that's going wrong and completely fall to pieces. And that's a big reason why a lot of us suffer from depression.

Homework

What I'd really encourage you to do now is to come up with a list of reasons to love yourself that are in your control, independent of circumstances, and independent of what other people think of you.

As we've said, it's very important to be extremely mindful of the reasons why you ought to love yourself, because it will contribute to you being much better able to cope with adversity and to prevent it from plummeting you into depression. So set aside some time to create this list, and then keep reading and re-reading it so that you train your brain to love yourself for those healthy reasons.

Key takeaways from this chapter

1/ "Healthy" reasons to love ourselves include:

a) Our skills—i.e. things that we're good at;
b) Our personal qualities and characteristics.

2/ These reasons to love ourselves are healthy because they are:

a) In our control;
b) Independent of what other people think of us;
c) Independent of circumstances.

3/ Similarly, "unhealthy" reasons to love ourselves are reasons that are:

a) *Not* in our control;
b) *Not* independent of what other people think of us;
c) *Not* independent of circumstances.

4/ When we love ourselves for healthy reasons, we are much better able to weather adversity than we would be if we loved ourselves for unhealthy reasons.

CHAPTER 4
Common Cause of People's Depression #3:
Anger

"Holding onto anger is like drinking poison and expecting someone else to die. The only person it hurts is you."

If you've read my *Depression is a Liar*, then you'll be very familiar with a girl called Chanel. We dated for four or five months, over which time my feelings for her grew to the point where I envisioned marrying her one day and spending my life with her. But we broke up when I realised that the whole time we'd been going out, she'd been cheating on me with one of my best friends. When I found out, I was furious. I was heartbroken. And to make matters even worse, I later heard that she began spreading the lie that I'd raped her.

In the aftermath of all this, I was not only very hurt, but also enraged. Remember in the previous chapter, where I said that one of the reasons why I love myself and one of the things that I take a lot of pride in is the fact that I'm kind to people, that I'm compassionate, and that I act with integrity? Well, to hear all of that being called into question . . . to hear someone say that I'd been acting in such a vile and despicable way—particularly somebody who I loved and who I thought felt the same way about me, and somebody who had already betrayed me by cheating on me with one of my best friends––it was absolutely devastating. I was horribly distraught. And like I've said, above all else, I was disturbingly mad.

To be completely honest with you, I was so angry with her that I wanted to kill her.

Of course, I did no such thing. I knew that the best revenge in such cases is living well, and I knew that I needed to forget about Chanel and move on in order to do so, because as we opened this chapter by saying, holding onto anger is like drinking poison and expecting someone else to die. The only person it hurts is us.

And for this reason, it is in *our* best interest to forgive those who have done harm to us.

Why should we forgive someone who's hurt us badly?

I understand if you're objecting to this notion right now. I understand if you're thinking:

I don't want to forgive the people who've wronged me! They really screwed me over! I hate them! The last thing they deserve from me is forgiveness!

I get it. I've felt that way too. But what I learned in time was that the reason why it's in our best interest to forgive the people who've wronged us is because it gives *us* peace—and this is exactly why I chose to forgive Chanel. Did she deserve it? I don't know, and I don't care. Whether or not she deserved it is completely irrelevant. Again, I chose to forgive her so that I could gain closure and move on with my life, because I knew that if I didn't—if I instead held onto the anger that I was feeling for her forever—it would just continue to poison me. And after all, Chanel had already hurt me once . . . I didn't want to give her the power to hurt me again.

The second point I want to make about forgiveness is that when we choose to forgive someone, it doesn't mean that we're all of a sudden condoning what that person did to hurt us. Again, we're forgiving them because it gives *ourselves* peace—and it's entirely possible to do so while at the same time holding the belief that what that person did to us was terribly wrong.

The third point I want to make is that choosing to forgive someone doesn't mean that the pain and anger we feel towards that person is going to immediately disappear. It takes time for anger to fade and for our pain to heal. However, when we forgive the people who have wronged us, it allows the healing process to finally begin.

Lastly, I'd like to stress the point that forgiveness does not have to lead to any sort of reunion with the person who's wronged us. In fact, I think that often the best way to forgive someone is to do so privately in our head. For the record, I never told Chanel that I forgave her. In fact, I haven't spoken to her since a couple of days after I caught her cheating on me, way back on New Year's Eve of 2007. I think there are some people like Chanel that we're better off without—but that doesn't mean that we can't forgive those people to free ourselves from the anger we feel toward them.

I'll close this chapter by saying that I know the act of forgiving someone who's wronged us is difficult. I know it may seem counterintuitive. And, I know that it's often the last thing in the world that we feel like doing. But I can promise you from experience that if you choose to do so, you are going to feel infinitely better as a result. You are going to feel so much more at peace with yourself, and so much more at peace with the world. You're going to feel as if a huge weight has been lifted off you. And as a result, you're going to feel much less depressed.

Key takeaways from this chapter

1/ Holding onto anger is like drinking poison and expecting someone else to die—the only person it hurts is us. For this reason, it is in our best interest to forgive all the people who have wronged us.

2/ Whether or not a person who has wronged us deserves our forgiveness is irrelevant. It's in our best interest to forgive such people because doing so gives us peace, and allows us to move on with our lives.

3/ Choosing to forgive someone who has wronged us does not mean that we condone what they did to us.

4/ Choosing to forgive someone who has wronged us does not mean that the pain and anger we feel toward that person is going to immediately disappear. However, choosing to forgive that person will allow the healing process to begin.

5/ Forgiving someone who has wronged us does not need to lead to a reunion with that person. Often the best way to forgive someone is to do so privately in our head.

CHAPTER 5
Common Cause of People's Depression #4:
Not allowing gratitude to co-exist with our pain

"Gratitude unlocks the fullness of life. It turns what we do into enough, and more. It turns denial into acceptance, chaos to order, confusion to clarity. It can turn a meal into a feast, a house into a home, a stranger into a friend."
Melody Beattie

When I say that a common cause of depression is not allowing gratitude to co-exist with our pain, I'm definitely not implying that we're not entitled to suffer from depression because there are people worse off than us, or that if we just realised how lucky we were, we wouldn't be depressed. No-one has the right to diminish or trivialise any pain we may be feeling, and just because someone may be worse off than us, it certainly doesn't mean that we're not allowed to hurt or suffer from depression ourselves. What I *am* saying, however, is that in order to recover from depression, it's extremely important to maintain an accurate perspective, and feel gratitude *in addition* to any pain we may be feeling.

How having gratitude saved my life

In hindsight, having gratitude was such a driving force in my recovery from depression because it gave me *perspective*. And we need to have perspective for two very important reasons:

1/ When we have perspective, we appreciate everything much more than someone who doesn't. As a result, we're much less depressed.

2/ Perspective gives us the positive attitude we need to be able to navigate our way through our depression and find the light at the end of the tunnel.

Let me now illuminate these two points by talking about how I personally came to be so conscious of what I'm grateful for, and how having gratitude quite literally saved my life.

When I finished high school at the end of 2006, I was lucky enough to be offered a scholarship to study Commerce/Law at Sydney University, and as such, found myself one evening at the scholarship presentation dinner. A couple of my high school teachers were invited to attend, and at some point, one of them said to me:

'You've been blessed with so much, Danny. You've been brought up in a wonderful neighbourhood; you're surrounded by a loving, supportive family; and you've got the opportunity and the ability to do anything you want to in life.'

Mr Williams then paused for a moment.

'I hope you use your blessings for good,' he said. 'I hope you always do charity work, and I hope you always try to help people. Remember, Danny: to whom much is given, much is expected.'

That notion really stuck in my mind, and in time, inspired me to volunteer for a month at an underprivileged school in Cusco, Peru.

At that point, I was amidst the thick of my depression, having been suffering for six months or a year; but when I arrived in Cusco and started witnessing some of the tragedies that were taking place there, it made me realise how lucky I truly was. To quote à section from *Depression is a Liar*:

Before I went to Cusco, I'd never been to a place where 56% of the population lived on less than US$1 a day, where 85% of children never attended high school, where the school dropout rate was 40%, where the unemployment rate was 42%, where the underemployment rate was 74%, where the literacy rate was 18%, where the infant mortality rate was 5%, and where the average life expectancy was 41 years.

I'd never met any children who wore the same World Vision clothes to school every day.

I'd never been to a school where not a single kid was fat, nor had I ever been called fat by anyone else, which is what some of the children thought the volunteers were because we weren't bone-skinny.

I'd never had 10 year olds try to sell me cigarettes on the street at two in the morning on a school night to help support their family.

I'd never been too embarrassed to tell someone I had a swimming pool in my backyard, like I was when my host family—who lived in a flat barely larger than my living room—had asked me to describe my home to them.

I'd never lived in a place where only ice-cold water came out of the taps, meaning that I had to heat it with a kettle and use a bucket and cup to shower.

I'd never seen villages of houses that didn't have any windows and were made out of mud bricks, much less had I helped build chimneys out of bamboo for said houses so that smoke wouldn't suffocate the air when the families cooked over a fire.

I'd never been to a place where all the adults looked 20 years older than their actual age, and where people as young as 30 had dry and wrinkled skin.

I'd never met a kid who grabbed other peoples' crotches and stuck his fingers up their bums during a school yard game of dodge ball.

'Why does he do that?' one of the volunteers asked.

'Because . . . he gets sexually abused at home.'

'By who?'

The volunteer manager released a painful sigh.

'By his father.'

We were all flabbergasted.

'How come . . . how come no-one's reported it?'

'We have.'

'And?'

He sighed again.

'The police . . . it's not like in your country. There's so much corruption . . . it's not like in your country.'

'But surely something can be done about it?'

'I'm afraid not.'

Seeing this poverty, this exploitation, this corruption, this perversion; waking up every morning and staring it in the face . . . it helped me think about my own set of worries in a different light.

Yeah, I do suffer from depression, I remember thinking, *but I'm still really lucky. I'm so fortunate to live in a safe country, to be surrounded by a supportive family, and to have the opportunity to*

do whatever I want with my life. So while I'm not without my problems, I'm also not without some incredible blessings.

Having such a high degree of gratitude sitting beside my pain helped give me a different perspective about my depression, and this perspective continued to develop in the months and years that followed. When I got back to Sydney, I started volunteering with a charity that supported battered women, and learning about the hardship that they go through further reinforced my belief that while I did have depression, I was still an extremely lucky person in many other ways. This gratitude then led me to co-found The Open Skies Foundation at the start of 2010, a non-profit organisation that aimed to create sustainable change in Third World Communities.

'But Danny, you're deeply suffering yourself right now,' the people close to me would say. 'You're going through one of the worst bouts of depression you've ever been through. Why would you now, of all times, decide to found a charity?'

And they were right—I *was* going through an awful time myself. Yet in spite of that, I still felt immensely fortunate for all the *good* things that I knew existed in my life alongside my despair—and this gratitude ignited an urge in me to want to help others who weren't bestowed with the privileges that I'd always known. And perhaps ironically, it was this commitment to helping other people that ended up saving my life several months later—as you can see from this passage from *Depression is a Liar*:

Woke up feeling ghastly. Dad drove me to uni for my exam. Silence all the way.

He dropped me off. I dragged myself to the exam room in a soulless, debilitated shuffle. When I got there I fell to the floor, sat slumped against the wall. My classmates talked to me, asked me questions, but still . . . nothing.

We got called in.

'Ten minutes reading time, starting now,' the announcer said.

I tried to read. I understood the words on their own, but put together they made no sense. I flicked through the exam. Not much of it did.

The exam itself began. I reread questions I knew I'd studied for, but in the moment the answers were a blur. I felt like I was in a trance. The world seemed a black hole. A vacuum of agony. I couldn't see any escape. The only possible salvation seemed death.

I scribbled down a few answers before the end of the exam.

'How did you go?' one of my friends asked. But I just shook my head and shuffled spiritlessly away.

I pulled myself into the streets. It was pouring down with rain. I had no idea what to do next. Should I go home? Go back to uni and study? Go to a coffee shop? Call a friend? Get smashed at a bar? Every possibility seemed brutally unbearable. The only one that didn't was killing myself. As you know, I'd always thought suicide was selfish, because even though it might've given me peace, I knew it would've left my family in ruins. But right then, on what was, unquestionably, the worst day of my life to date, I started to think that maybe I was wrong. I started to think that perhaps I'd been too narrow-minded.

Because I swear, *I vividly remember thinking,* if my family knew how depressed I am right now . . . if they could comprehend the gut-wrenching severity of the pain I'm in . . . I swear they'd want me to put myself out of my misery. I swear they'd want me to end it all and finally be free.

It was a dangerous revelation.

Does this mean I can die now? *I thought.* Guilt-free and with my family's blessing?

I stopped walking, let the rain pound down on top of me.

Can I do it? Can I really kill myself? Jump in front of a speeding car and join the rest of the road toll casualties?

I stood at a right angle to the road, watched the cars zooming by.

Is this really it? Can I really end it all right here?

My mind was a warzone. So much conflict. But eventually there emerged a definite answer.

No.

I can't do it.

It's the answer I'd always reached, but this time, the reason was different.

It wasn't for me.

It wasn't even for my family.

It was for those less fortunate than me.

Regardless of how depressed I feel right now, *I thought,* I know that I've been tremendously blessed: with a loving, supportive family; with First World privileges; and with the opportunity and the ability to do whatever I want to in life. Regardless of how I feel right now, I have had a lot bestowed upon me, and I have to use my good fortune to help others who aren't as immensely privileged as I am. If I kill myself, Open Skies will disband. All the charity work I'd planned on doing will never get done. I'd be abandoning all the people I have the capacity to help. And no matter how much pain I'm in I just can't do that. To whom much is given, much is expected. I can't kill myself. Not now, not ever.

I felt it so strongly, with such paramount force that it couldn't be doubted. It was as if it was a calling, a message from God in my hour of need:

I put you on this earth for a reason, Danny. You can't leave it. There's so much work that you need to do . . .

So I stepped away from the road. I called my mum.

'Hello?'

'Ma . . .' I croaked.

'Danny? Are you alright?'

I murmured something inaudible.

'Danny?' she panicked. 'Is everything OK?'

'Come and get me . . . please. Wynyard.'

I met her there, crawled into the car, muttered in broken sentences what happened.

'Danny, we would never want you to kill yourself!' she stressed. 'Never, ever, ever, ever! Suicide is a permanent solution to a temporary problem! You know that, don't you?'

I eventually managed to nod my head. From the corner of my barely opened eye, I saw Mum fighting back tears as she tried to drive through the rain. At some point she pulled over to call my dad. She talked to him while I sat motionless in the front seat.

After a long time, she finally hung up.

'Danny . . .' she murmured. 'Danny we think . . . we think it's time you be admitted to hospital.'

She paused solemnly.

'What do you think?'

I just wanted to get better. I was so tired of feeling sick and I just wanted to get better.

'OK,' I managed to say. 'I'll go to hospital.'

As you can see, gratitude really did save my life, because if it wasn't for being so conscious of how lucky I really am, then I may not have

had anything else to stop me from jumping in front of those speeding cars.

Since that day, I've done a lot more charity work through Open Skies, various other organisations, and most recently, as a mental health advocate—and in the course of doing so, I've seen some absolutely heartbreaking things.

I've met seven year old Cambodian girls who have to beg on the streets to get their food because their parents are too busy gambling and getting high to feed them. Sometimes they also have to beg to get food for their parents, and if they don't get enough, their parents beat them.

I've met girls who started being sexually abused when they were three.

I've met refugees as young as 10 who've lost their entire families at sea when they tried to come to Australia.

I've met suicidal 14 year old kids who've been kicked out of home and forced to live on the streets because their parents "don't believe in mental illness" and are sick of them being "drama queens".

This is just the tip of the iceberg—I could go on forever with these stories—but the point to note is that witnessing all of these tragedies has helped me realise how fortunate I really am, and filled me with gratitude for all the privileges that I've been blessed with. Like I've said, having such a high degree of gratitude is the reason I'm still alive today, because it prevented me from jumping in front of those speeding cars; however, it's also been the saving grace of my life for two other very important reasons.

Firstly, it kept me positive throughout my entire fight with depression, which allowed me to navigate my way through it and beat it in the end.

Secondly, not only did it lead me to beat my depression, but it also led me to be happier than I ever thought I could be, because it's

made me really, truly appreciate my life. As a result, I now get so much more enjoyment out of everything than I otherwise would.

For example, because I know how lucky I am to be able to walk peacefully down the street without having to worry about being assaulted or shot—something that's commonplace in many war-ravaged countries—I can derive a lot of pleasure, enjoyment and appreciation from an act that's often taken for granted like strolling down the road to a coffee shop. It's the same with other simple pleasures like having lunch at a nice café with a friend, flicking on the T.V. and watching a basketball game, or lying in the sun at the beach—because I'm cognisant of how lucky I am to be able to do seemingly little things like this when so many other people in the world can't, I can really appreciate them, and thus get so much more enjoyment out of them than I otherwise would.

I'm telling you: the more gratitude you have in your life, the happier you will be, because you're going to appreciate everything so much more than you otherwise would.

And you *do* have reasons to be grateful.

I don't know anything about you, but since you have access to a computer and can afford to buy this book, you have a lot more than hundreds of millions of people in the world.

Just to reiterate, I'm not saying this to belittle any pain you may be feeling or to make you feel guilty for suffering from depression. Like I said at the start of this chapter, just because there may be people in the world who are worse off than you, it certainly doesn't mean that you're not entitled to your grief. Instead, what I'm saying is that in order to beat your depression and become the happy person that you want to be, it's vital that you maintain an accurate perspective about your life, and allow an appropriate level of gratitude to co-exist with your anguish.

What can we do to have more gratitude in our lives?

Having gratitude is so central to being happy that it's become a field of study in and of itself, leading to books and articles being written, studies being undertaken and apps being developed to help us become more grateful and conscious of all the beauty, joy and pleasure that exists in our lives. Having been a student of gratitude for several years now, I'd like to share with you some of the things that have helped me become more grateful over the years, and some of the tips, tools and tricks I know have worked for others.

Help someone less fortunate than ourselves

Like I've said, the main reason I'm so grateful is because I've done so much volunteer work, and have thus met countless people whose lives are much more trying that mine. If you're in a position to do so, I recommend travelling to a Third World country to do some too, and to witness how people much less fortunate than ourselves live.

If that's not feasible, then I'd recommend doing something more locally—like volunteering at your local homeless shelter or at your closest children's hospital. Not only will this help give you perspective and cause you to feel more grateful about all the positive things in your life, but there are also few things in the world that are more uplifting and more rewarding to do than to offer your time to help other people less fortunate than yourself. It's such a wonderfully gratifying thing to do—just watching a little kid's face light up when you give them a yoyo, or having someone reach for your hand and say "thank-you, you've helped me, you've had a positive impact on my life" is one of the most beautiful feelings you can experience.

If you don't have the time to do volunteer work but you do have the money to be able to help someone less fortunate than yourself, then becoming a donor—regardless of how much or how little you donate—can make a huge difference to someone's life and heighten your gratitude for your own good fortune. You could do something like sponsor a hungry child through World Vision, or, if you have a soft spot for mental health, you could donate to an organisation like NAMI, SANE or Beyond Blue.

Keep a gratitude journal

Every night before you go to bed, write down five things that you're grateful for—either things that you're thankful that you were able to do that day, or things that you're thankful for in general. For example:

- I'm grateful for having been able to eat my favourite meal for dinner tonight.

- I'm grateful for being able to spend time with my family today.
- I'm grateful for living in a safe, beautiful country.
- I'm grateful that today was a sunny day, and that I got to enjoy it by being able to take a stroll in the park.
- I'm grateful for my partner.

See how easy it is? It doesn't take long, and it can really help you focus on all the positive things in your life. In fact, studies have shown that gratitude exercises such as this result in increased alertness, enthusiasm, determination, optimism and energy, in addition to—you guessed it—decreased levels of depression.

I've personally found it immensely beneficial to keep a gratitude diary in this way, however leading gratitude researcher Robert Emmons suggests in his book Gratitude Works! that there's an even more effective way to keep a gratitude journal: instead of picking five things that you're grateful for each day, pick one thing and write five reasons why you're grateful for it. For example, I'm grateful for my brother because he:

- Makes me laugh.
- Is always honest with me.
- Always makes the most of the time we spend together.
- Is always there when I need him.
- Helps me relax and enjoy my life.

I like both methods, so these days, I mix it up—sometimes I do one and sometimes I do the other. I'd recommend giving both a try and seeing what works best for you.

Lastly, in terms of how to logistically keep your gratitude journal, you can of course use a regular diary, or, you can use the immensely popular Gratitude Journal app.

Key takeaways from this chapter

1/ Being grateful for all the wonderful things in our lives is very important because it gives us perspective, which is essential to our wellbeing because:

a) When we have perspective, we appreciate everything so much more than we otherwise would;

b) Perspective gives us the positive attitude we need to be able to navigate our way through our depression, and find the light at the end of the tunnel.

2/ A great way to inject more gratitude into our lives is to:

a) Do volunteer work;
b) Keep a gratitude journal.

CHAPTER 6
Common Cause of People's Depression #5:
Victimising ourselves

"As long as you think that the cause of your problem is "out there"—as long as you think that anyone or anything is responsible for your suffering—the situation is hopeless. It means that you are forever in the role of victim, that you're suffering in paradise."
Byron Katie

This is a really important topic, because unfortunately, many people I interact with who suffer from depression constantly victimise themselves. It's a very human thing to do. Whenever something goes wrong in our lives, often our natural reaction is to think:

Why is this happening to me? Nobody else I know has to deal with this! I'm a good person . . . I don't deserve this! This is so unfair! Why do bad things always happen to me and me only?

However, while it's easy to do, victimising ourselves is a very unhealthy habit to get into, because if we do victimise ourselves, it's almost impossible to recover from depression.

Here's the cold hard reality: bad things happen, and feeling sorry for ourselves won't get us anywhere. When we are struck by adversity or when we suffer from depression, instead of complaining

and acting like a victim, we need to confront our problems, resolve them, and then move on from them.

When I say this, please understand that I'm not trying to be dismissive of your hardship or to trivialise it in any way, nor am I coming at this from the perspective of a person who's never experienced anything painful or heartbreaking. I've been through my fair share of problems, too. I haven't told you before, but when I was 15, my dream was to be a professional basketball player. I was pouring everything I had into achieving it, but then I severely injured my knee, and whatever chance I had was gone. A couple of years later, I had that disastrous relationship with Chanel, and then a few months after that I started suffering from depression, which over the next four years led to alcoholism, drug abuse, medicine-induced psychosis, near-suicide attempts and multiple hospitalisations. No matter what I was going through, however, I made a point of never victimising myself, because I knew that doing so would lead me to feel bitter, spiteful and even more miserable. Instead, I chose to face my problems, resolve them, and then move on from them—and it's this approach I really believe we need to take if we don't want our *temporary* problems to turn into *permanent* problems.

At the end of the day, this is exactly what victimising ourselves does: turn adversity that we can overcome in time into adversity that will plague us forever, by changing our focus from *what can I do to resolve my problems?* into *Why do bad things always happen to me? Life is so unfair! I don't deserve this at all!* And the

problem with this latter approach is that it doesn't lead us to take the proactive steps that we need to take in order to overcome our hardship. Rather, it leads us to wallow in our misery, and wallowing in our misery is a sure-fire way to stay trapped in depression forever.

What can we do to feel less like a victim?

Each of the following practices are ones I commonly employ to this day to help prevent me from feeling sorry for myself whenever something in my life doesn't go according to plan.

Focus on moving forwards

Like I've said, when adversity strikes us, I firmly believe that the best thing we can do for ourselves is to confront our problems, resolve them, and then move on from them. If this is out mindset, then when we fall on hard times, we're so busy trying to deal with our problems and move on from them that we don't have time to feel sorry for ourselves.

Take responsibility

When something goes wrong in our lives, I also believe it's in our best interest to analyse the situation, take responsibility for all the mistakes we've made, and learn as much as we can from the experience to try and prevent it from ever occurring again. This approach is the opposite of the "blaming everybody else" approach, which is so often at the root cause of self-victimisation.

Let go of anger

Taking the steps that we need to take in order to let go of anger once again shifts our approach from "blaming everybody else" to being focused on moving forwards. Looking back, I can see that it's because I worked so hard to forgive Chanel that I didn't victimise myself when everything went awry with her.

Gratitude, gratitude, gratitude

When I injured my knee, one of the main things that stopped me from victimising myself was reminding myself of all the blessings in my life, even though my dream was shattered. Because I had gratitude sitting beside my pain, I was able to say to myself:

OK, this is really heartbreaking, but on the bright side, I'm still only 15 years old. What happened is devastating, yes, but it hardly means my life is over. I'm fortunate enough to go to a very good school where I'm able to receive a great education, so even though I can no longer be a professional basketball player, if I make the most of the wonderful opportunities still available to me, I'll be able to recover from this setback, and go on to live a happy life.

Key takeaways from this chapter

1/ Victimising ourselves turns our *temporary* problems into *permanent* problems, since it changes our focus from *what can I do to resolve this problem?* to *Why do bad things always happen to me? Life is so unfair! I don't deserve this at all!* This latter approach doesn't lead us to take the proactive steps that we need to take in order to overcome our hardship. Instead, it leads us to wallow in it, and wallowing in our problems is a sure-fire way to stay trapped in our depression.

2/ When we're hit with adversity, we can take various steps to reduce and eliminate the "I'm a victim" feeling by:

a) Focusing on moving forwards;

b) Analysing what went wrong, taking responsibility for any mistakes we may have made, and learning what we can from the experience so that we can minimise the chance of it happening again;

c) Working to let go of the anger that we feel towards the situation;

d) Working at being more grateful for all of the good things that exist in our lives—even though we're going through adversity at the moment.

CHAPTER 7
Common Cause of People's Depression #6:
Not being surrounded by the "right" people . . . or even worse, being surrounded by "toxic" people

"You are the average of the five people you spend the most time with."
Jim Rohn

Author and motivational speaker Jim Rohn once remarked that we are the average of the five people who we spend the most time with. And I think he's right. As you've probably experienced yourself, who you surround yourself with affects the way you think, the way you feel, and the decisions you make.

For this reason, in order to recover from depression and become the happy people that we want to be, it's critically important that we surround ourselves with the "right" people and distance ourselves from the "wrong" people.

However, this then raises the question: *How are we supposed to know who the "right" people and who the "wrong" people are?*

This is something I really used to struggle with, so I asked a psychologist for his advice. Below is an exercise he taught me to do which, despite its simplicity, really worked wonders. I'll lay it out like a high school science experiment, just for a bit of fun.

Aim

To figure out who the "right" people and who the "wrong" people to surround ourselves with are.

Materials needed

- An A4 piece of paper;
- A pen;
- A person who's ready to learn and improve their surroundings (that's us!).

Method

1/ Draw a mind-map connected to a centre circle that asks, "what do I value in a friend?"

2/ Around the circle, write down the characteristics or personality traits that you appreciate in a friend. For example, loyalty, kindness, or someone who's down to earth. Let me emphasise that it is very important that you don't rush this part. Make sure you really think about what you value in a friend so that what you write down accurately reflects your true feelings. The benefits of this exercise is in getting this section "right"—so if you rush it and jot down characteristics or personality traits in a friend that *don't* correctly reflect your true feelings, then this exercise won't help you achieve the results that it can.

Conclusions

1/ Everyone who possesses the characteristics and personality traits that we've identified as valuing in a friend are the "right" people for us to surround ourselves with. As a result, we want to

make a deliberate effort to surround ourselves with these people, because we're in all likelihood going to have really positive, healthy relationships with them.

2/ On the other hand, those who do not possess the characteristics and personality traits that we've identified as valuing in a friend are the "wrong" people for us to surround ourselves with. For this reason, it's in our best interest to distance ourselves from such people, because we're in all likelihood going to have negative relationships with them.

~~~

I know this exercise sounds simple. I know this exercise may sound corny. But it can really work if you take the time to do it properly. Like I said, the value of it comes in taking the time to identify what you truly desire in a friend, because it's this level of self-awareness that is ultimately going to lead you to make good, healthy decisions about who you choose to spend your time with.

Toxic people

Another thing that's worth noting is that there are certain traits that make up some people which are outright toxic, and if we surround ourselves with people who have such characteristics, it's likely to compromise our happiness. Over the years, I've talked to thousands of people who have depression, and one of the biggest triggers for
~~~

many sufferers is that they have toxic people in their lives who exhibit some of the following traits.

1/ **They're judgmental.** Instead of being supportive, some people are critically judgmental. For example, if you suffer from depression, then choosing to see a therapist is an excellent decision to make. However, a judgmental person may condemn you for that. They may think, *oh, so-and-so is seeing a psychologist . . . that means they must be really weird! That means they must be crazy!* And we never want to be surrounded by people like that.

2/ **Jealousy.** Supportive people will celebrate with us when we have a success, but jealous people are likely to try and drag us down instead. Those are people we're definitely better off without.

3/ **People who don't believe in us.** Again, people who don't believe in us are the opposite of supportive, and it's not in our best interest to surround ourselves with such people.

4/ **People who take their anger and frustration out on us when something goes wrong in their life.** There are certain people who will constantly treat us like garbage whenever something is bothering them, even if what's bothering them has nothing to do with us. We deserve better.

5/ **People who bring out the worst in us.** For example, if you're a recovering alcoholic and you're trying to stop drinking, then a supportive person will respect your decision and encourage you to lay off the bottle. On the other hand, a toxic person will suggest that you go to the pub together and "just have a few rounds".

6/ **People who try to change us from the person we are into the person that they want us to be.** We are all unique, and if someone tries to trample on our individuality and turn us into someone we're not, then they're not a good person for us to be around. It's really hard to be happy when someone's forcing their beliefs about how we should look, act or think down our throats.

What if I'm not sure about someone?

We can use everything we've learned so far in this chapter to help us figure out who the "right" and who the "wrong" and/or "toxic" people to surround ourselves with are. However, there may be times when we're still not quite sure about a particular person, which can sometimes happen when they possess a few of the characteristics we value in a friend, but they also possess some of the toxic traits we want nothing to do with. In such an instance, it helps to ask ourselves the following question, which can serve to give us a definitive answer.

After I've spent time with that person, how do I feel?

If you feel in a positive mood after you see them, then that's a "good" person for you to spend your time with. However, as you probably know from experience, there are certain people who will repeatedly leave you feeling down after you've engaged with them. Maybe you find that your confidence is lower because they don't believe in you. Maybe you feel exhausted because they dump their problems on you all the time. Maybe you feel angry because every time you have some good news, instead of celebrating it with you, they are jealous, spiteful, and try to minimise your success. Whatever it may be, here's the critical point to note: if you continuously feel down after spending time with someone, then it's not in your best interest to be around that person.

As the saying goes, throughout our lives,
we will constantly meet angels and devils,

and we only know who is who *after* we've met them.

What if the toxic person in our lives is a family member? Or, someone we've known for a really long time?

Being family does not preclude someone from being a toxic person. Just because someone is a parent, sibling, in-law, cousin, aunt or uncle, it doesn't strip them of their power to have a very negative impact on our lives. Accordingly, if we have a family member who either exhibits a lot of the toxic traits we've talked about or who does not have the characteristics that we value in a friend, then I think it behoves us to distance ourselves from that person. I know it can be difficult. I know it's not always practical to cut them completely out of our lives. However, I still think it's worth putting as much space between them and us as we can. At the end of the day, our happiness is too important to have them compromise it.

The same goes for someone we've been friends with for a very long time. They can be toxic too, and sometimes there comes a time in our relationship with that person when we have to move on. Once again, our happiness is too important to have them poison it.

Key takeaways from this chapter

1/ People who possess the characteristics and personality traits that we value in a friend are the "right" people for us to surround ourselves with, because we're likely to have very positive, healthy relationships with those people. On the other hand, people who do not possess the characteristics and personality traits that we value in a friend are the "wrong" people for us to surround ourselves with, because we're likely to have very negative, toxic relationships with those people.

2/ People who are judgmental, who are jealous, who don't believe in us, who take their anger and frustration out on us when something doesn't go right in their life, who bring out the worst in us, who try to change us, and most importantly, who leave us feeling down after we've spent time with them are toxic people for us to surround ourselves with.

3/ Just because someone is family or someone we've known for a very long time, it does not preclude them from being a toxic person.

CHAPTER 8
Common Cause of People's Depression #7:
Being a prisoner of what other people think

"If you care about what other people think, you will always be their prisoner."
Lao Tzu

Judging by all the emails I get, I know that being held captive by what other people think is a huge trigger for a lot of people's depression. Now, I would never say that we should completely ignore what everyone else thinks and never take into consideration anything they say, because it's undoubtedly good to listen to others and be mindful of their thoughts. However, I do believe that we should stop short of becoming *prisoners* of their opinions, because that can lead us to do things against our better judgment, or to do things that aren't in our own best interest—and this can certainly lead to depression.

In what ways is it possible to be prisoners of what other people think of us?

We can be held captive by what other people think of us in two main ways.

1/ By defining ourselves by what others think of us

Remember when we talked about the importance of basing our love for ourselves on reasons that are *in our control*, that are *independent of what other people think of us*, and that are *independent of circumstances*? And, remember when we said that when we *don't* do this—i.e. when we instead base our love for ourselves on what other people think of us—then we give those people so much power over our happiness?

Speaking from the heart, I truly believe that one of the reasons why I'm so happy today is because I really don't mind what other people think of me. And if you remember from earlier on, this is because I don't base my love for myself on what other people think of me. If people think I'm a freak because I used to suffer from depression, then I don't mind. If they don't like something I write somewhere, I don't mind. I don't need their validation to be able to love myself, because I have a whole bunch of reasons to love myself that are *independent* of what other people think of me. And this is really important, because when we love ourselves for reasons that

are independent of what others think of us, we can free ourselves from their opinions, and as a result, greatly ease our depression.

2/ By letting what others think of us govern the decisions we make

We are also prisoners of what other people think of us when we allow them to govern the decisions we make, which can be a major problem for people with depression. For example, I've spoken to countless people who've told me something along the lines of:

'I know that seeking help is a good idea, but what will everyone think of me if I do? They might think I'm crazy . . . and that scares me. So I haven't sought help.'

In this case, letting what other people may think of us dictate the decisions we make is having a detrimental effect on our health and happiness, since seeking help is vital to recovering from depression (just for the record by the way, chances are that not many people—if anyone—are going to think you're "crazy" for seeing a psychologist).

Letting what other people think of us govern the decisions we make can also harm us in many other aspects of our lives. For example, it can cause us to pursue a career we don't really enjoy, get romantically involved with someone we don't really love, end a romantic relationship with someone we *do* really love, waste money on something that we don't really want, or cause us to make practically any other bad decision you can think of.

I understand how scary it can sometimes be to follow our hearts and go against what other people may think of us, but the truth is that if we don't, then we will end up being the person that *other people* want us to be, instead of the person that *we* want to be.

You might be thinking:

OK, I get that in theory, and I agree, but how do I actually go about emotionally freeing myself from what other people think of me so that I'm then able to make decisions that aren't dictated by what they think?

Well, here's a notion that's always helped me.

When trying to free ourselves from what other people think of us, it helps to remember a line from Dr Seuss: *"those who matter don't mind and those who mind don't matter"*.

I really do believe this. The "right" people are going to be supportive of the decisions we make, and if someone's not, then like we said in the previous chapter, they're probably not a person we want to spend time with anyway. In fact, this is something I can specifically recall my psychologist explaining to me before I released my memoir *Depression is a Liar* in 2013.

'So Danny, how've you been feeling?' he asked when I arrived.

'Yeah, really good on the whole. But I've been a bit nervous lately about publishing my memoir. I mean, hardly anyone knows that I used to suffer from depression . . . so what are they going to say when they find out I used to? And what are they going to say when they find out that it led to alcoholism, drug abuse, medicine-induced psychosis, near-suicide attempts and multiple hospitalisations? What if some of my friends read my book, conclude that I'm a freak, and then decide they don't want to be friends with me anymore?'

'I don't think anyone is going to think that,' my psychologist said. 'But even if a few people do, I don't think it really matters.'

I was shocked.

'Huh? How can you say that it doesn't matter?'

My psychologist smiled at me gently.

'When you release your memoir, Danny, there are going to be a lot of people who find it inspiring, uplifting and encouraging—and dare I say it, I think there are going to be some people who find it life-saving. However, you may also get some people who can't deal with it, and for that reason, choose to distance themselves from you. But let me ask you this: if someone chooses to distance themselves from you because they don't like your past or because they think you're a "freak", as you put it, then do you think you'd ever be able to have a good relationship with that person anyway?'

I thought about it for a few moments.

'No,' I eventually said. 'I guess not.'

'Would you even want to be friends with them?'

I considered that question for another few moments before shaking my head.

'No.'

'So then why would you care if a few people think like that after reading your memoir? Those who matter don't mind, and those who mind don't matter, remember?'

I really took that advice to heart, and ever since that conversation, I've never worried about what people think of me (just for the record, though, almost everyone I know was really supportive when they read my memoir—no-one called me a "freak" or anything like that, and I realised that I needn't have worried so much about people judging me. I think that's because most people appreciate that we're all battling something—but that's a different topic for another day).

Key takeaways from this chapter

1/ When we become prisoners of what other people think of us, it hurts us in two main ways:

a) By leading us to do things against our better judgment;
b) By leading us to do things that aren't in our own best interests.

2/ To free ourselves from what other people think of us, we want to:

a) Make sure that we love ourselves for reasons that are *independent* of what other people think of us;
b) Remember that those who matter don't mind, and those who mind don't matter.

CHAPTER 9
Common Cause of People's Depression #8:
Forgetting that we're only a part— and often only a very small part— of everyone else's world

"It's not about you. It's about them."
Clint Eastwood

Let me start this chapter by asking you a very important question:

When you have an interaction with someone that doesn't go according to plan, do you automatically assume that it's "your fault", or a consequence of one of your "personal failings"?

For example, you give your boss what you feel is a really good piece of work, but your boss isn't particularly enthusiastic about it––and as a result, you jump to the conclusion that your boss doesn't value your contribution at all, and that you're the weak link in the team.

Another example: your partner says they're not in the mood to have sex, and you jump to the conclusion that they're losing interest in you.

A third example: you go on a date with someone, and they don't call you for a second date—or, when you call them, they turn you down; as a result, you then jump to the conclusion that you're boring and unattractive.

Have you ever done something like this before?

I know I have. I've definitely exacerbated my depression in the past by convincing myself that the way someone else reacts to something I've done is a direct reflection on me.

But what I eventually learned is that when we think like this, what we're doing is completely ignoring the fact that the way someone reacts to us is not only a reflection on us, but also a reflection on *them* and *their* circumstances.

Let's go back to our examples.

Firstly, you give your boss what you feel is a really good piece of work, but they aren't enthusiastic about it—and as a result, you jump to the conclusion that your boss doesn't value your contribution, and that you're the weak link in the team. But, isn't it also possible that your boss was just in a bad mood because of something else that's entirely unrelated to you, and that their less-than-enthusiastic response to your work was just a projection of their prior irritation? And, if you're honest with yourself, haven't you done this before? Hasn't there been a time when your partner or your friend or your son or your daughter has come to you with something they're really excited about, but you brushed them off because you were angry or upset about something else?

Now let's turn to our second example, where your partner says they're not in the mood to have sex, and you then jump to the conclusion that they're losing interest in you. Now, anything's possible—maybe your partner *is* losing interest in you. But, isn't it also possible that they're just tired and not in the mood? Isn't it also possible that they're stressed out about something else, and for that reason, don't want to have sex? Isn't it also possible that they have something on early the next morning and just want to get some sleep? Aren't any of these reasons possible—in addition to a bunch of other reasons? And, hasn't there been a time when you've done the exact same thing yourself? Haven't you turned down having sex with your partner before not because you were no longer attracted

to them, but because of some other reason that's completely unrelated to them?

What about our third example, where a first date with someone doesn't lead to a second, so you jump to the conclusion that you're boring and unattractive. But let me ask you: isn't it also possible that the reason that person decided against going on a second date with you is not because they think you're boring and unattractive, but because they have a fear of commitment? Or because they met someone else? Or because they're coming off a recent break-up and on second thoughts, aren't ready to start dating another person yet? And again, haven't you at some point decided not to go on a second date with someone for a reason that has absolutely nothing to do with that person?

Here's the point: just because somebody has a less than positive response to something we do, we can't jump to negative conclusions about ourselves. When we do this, we are completely ignoring the fact that we are only a part—and often only a very small part—of that person's world. They—like us—have got a million things going on in their head that influence their decisions and their responses to certain events, and for this reason, it's entirely possible that when they have a less than positive reaction to

something we say or do, that it has absolutely nothing to do with us.

Knowing this, and being conscious of it, can be a very powerful, soothing concept that can eliminate a lot of our stress and significantly ease our depression.

Key takeaways from this chapter

1/ Just because somebody has a less than positive response to something we say or do, we can't jump to negative conclusions about ourselves. Doing so completely ignores the fact that we are only a part—and often only a very small part—of that person's world.

2/ For this reason, it's entirely possible that when someone else has a less than positive reaction to something we say or do, that it has absolutely nothing to do with us.

CHAPTER 10
Common Cause of People's Depression #9:
Living an unbalanced life

"Happiness is not a matter of intensity but of balance and order and rhythm and harmony."
Thomas Merton

In order for us to live a balanced life, we need to:

- Make sure that we're bringing in enough money to live off;
- Take care of our bodies by eating well, sleeping well and exercising frequently;
- Satisfy each of our core values (to refresh your memory, our core values are the things that mean the most to us in the world).

Sometimes it's OK to be temporarily unbalanced—for example, a student studying for his final year exams may choose to bury himself in his books and not see his friends for a few months, or pull an all-nighter cramming just before a test. However, if the student constantly lives this way—and if any of us continuously live an unbalanced life—it's likely to seriously trigger our depression.

What can we do to live a more balanced life?

Add structure to our days

It's certainly possible to live a very *un*structured yet balanced life, but it's been my observation that most of us are better at maintaining a balance when we make a point of scheduling time to do all the different things that we want to do. For example, if we don't set aside time to exercise, it often doesn't get done. However, if we schedule in our diaries to go to the gym at 6pm every Monday and Thursday, it's much more likely that we'll actually go.

Listen to our mind and body

If we're not doing enough of one thing or overdoing another, our mind or body will usually tell us. For example, if we constantly feel tired, then our body's trying to let us know that we need to sleep more. If we're feeling mentally drained and exhausted, then our mind's trying to warn us that we're working too hard.

Listen to our loved ones

For example, if our partner's complaining that we're always at work and never home, then they probably have a point.

Establish boundaries between "work time" and "leisure time"

It's good to work hard while we're in the office, but in the interest of living a balanced life, it's best if we leave our work at work. If we're always bringing files home or checking our smartphones to see if our boss has emailed, then we're making it very hard for ourselves to "switch off" and achieve a desirable work/life balance.

Let technology help us!

Because living a balanced life is something that so many of us struggle with, there are an abundance of apps that have been developed to help us do it. I recommend using one or more of the following, all of which are free or only cost a few dollars:

1/ iPlanSuccess: By allowing you to define your values, strengths and the ways you deal with being busy, this clever app helps you set realistic goals in order to achieve a better balance between your work and personal life.

2/ Cozi Family Organiser: This app lets you keep track of your family members' schedules so that you can know when they're free and thus set aside time to spend with them.

3/ SelfControl: This app lets you block access to distracting websites, your mail servers, or anything else on the internet for a pre-defined period of time. In addition to being a great productivity app, it will help you achieve a more balanced life by forcing you to take a time-out from work and do something else.

4/ Timer+: Like we've said, it's much easier to live a balanced life when we make a point of setting aside time to do each of the things that we want to do. This app helps you do that by allowing you to set a time limit on what you're doing so that you don't run

over time and miss out on doing something else. Multiple timers can be set at once, and alerts can be sent out even when the timer's running in the background.

5/ Crunch Time: The aim of this app is to provide busy users with an improved knowledge of how they spend their time, and to help them achieve a better balance between all their activities. Similar to the iPlanSuccess app, CrunchTime lets you set work-life balance goals in the areas of hours worked, sleep time, overtime worked, mood, weight and vacation taken, and awards you with an achievement badge every time a goal is met.

6/ Balanced: This app allows you to track the things you wish you did more often, and helps motivate you to do them again. Balanced will acknowledge when you achieve a goal by giving you positive feedback, will allow you to prioritise your activities in order of importance, will give you a list of 50 uplifting activities that you can do to improve your life, and much more.

7/ Life Balance: Marketed as personal coaching software, Life Balance dynamically adjusts your to-do list as you check off completed tasks to help you manage your time more efficiently.

8/ Wonderful Life Plan: This app allows you to set short, medium and long term goals and helps you keep track of whether or not you're achieving them.

If we suffer from depression, we also need to set aside time to …

We said before that in order to be happy and to live a balanced life, we need to make sure that we're satisfying each of our core values, in addition to making sure that we're bringing home enough money

to live off, and that we're taking care of our bodies by eating well, sleeping well and exercising frequently. This is 100% true, but if we suffer from depression, there's also one other critically important thing that we need to make time for in our lives.

> If we're suffering from depression, then part of living a balanced life involves doing the things that we need to do in order to recover from depression—such as seeing a therapist, reading self-help books such as this one, keeping mood diaries, and anything else that will help us understand what is causing us to feel depressed or help us to deal with that underlying cause.

While I haven't said this explicitly, it's certainly been implied that recovery from depression does *not* happen by being passive. It happens by confronting our demons, and then fighting like hell to try and beat them. Accordingly, in order to recover from depression, we need to make time to do whatever it takes for us to recover. We can't afford to be "too busy" to do such things.

Taking this into account, an amended list of things we need to do to live a balanced life if we suffer from depression would thus be:

- Making sure that we're bringing in enough money to live off;
- Taking care of our bodies by eating well, sleeping well and exercising frequently;

- Satisfying each of our core values;
- Doing whatever we need to do in order to recover from depression.

Key takeaways from this chapter

1/ In order to live a balanced life, we need to make sure that we're making enough money to live off; taking care of our bodies by eating well, sleeping well and exercising frequently; and satisfying each of our core values.

2/ To live a balanced life, it helps if we do the following:

a) Structure and plan our days;
b) Listen to our mind and body;
c) Listen to our loved ones;
d) Establish boundaries between our "work" time and our "leisure" time;
e) Use one or more of the many apps that exist for just this purpose.

3/ If we suffer from depression, then we also need to set aside time to do the things that we need to do in order to recover.

CHAPTER 11
Common Cause of People's Depression #10:
Perfectionism

"I'm a perfectionist. Sometimes I have to remind myself that it's OK if there are flaws here and there."

Tyra Banks

There's a lot to be said for being a perfectionist, as it pushes us to strive for excellence and to reach our true potential. However, it can also be a double-edged sword, which I learned at 19 when my perfectionism plunged me into depression. After two miserable years, I wound up in a psych ward, and quickly discovered how prevalent a problem it really was. Out of the 20 or so group therapy sessions I attended during that particular two week stay, the one on perfectionism drew by far the biggest crowd—the room was so packed that people had to bring in extra seats from their bedrooms, and latecomers had to sit on the floor. At the time, I was shocked. I had no idea that perfectionism was an Achilles heel for so many people. It always seemed to me to be such a good trait to have, so how was it that it had affected so many people so negatively?

As the session progressed, there emerged three main ways in which perfectionism seemed to harm people. We'll hash each of them out below, and talk about how we can stop these tendencies from triggering our depression.

> **Perfectionism can lead us to measure our self-worth in terms of how "perfectly" we achieve our goals—which can lead us to feel worthless, inadequate, like a failure, and to hate ourselves**

This was one of the main causes of my depression. Below is an excerpt from my memoir *Depression is a Liar*, where my psychologist summarised how my perfectionism triggered me and explained what I had to do to manage that trigger.

> *'You relentlessly seek excellence, Danny, and you always set extremely challenging goals and then throw yourself into achieving them. Being perfectionistically goal-driven like this is fine in and of itself, but the problem with you is that you measure your self-worth entirely in terms of whether or not you achieve these goals. If you don't achieve a goal that you set out to achieve-like getting a High Distinction average at university or getting your novel [that I'd been working on] published by a particular point in time, you hate yourself. You feel worthless and inadequate. You feel like a failure. And you feel this pain so intensely that you become suicidal.*
>
> *'You're human, Danny, and humans, by our very composition, are not perfect. Humans make mistakes. Humans don't always achieve their goals. You need to accept this, and not be so hard on yourself. You need to accept this, and be able to love yourself regardless. You need to be able to love yourself regardless of how you go in your uni exams and no matter what happens with your novel. Even if you fail every exam for the rest of*

your degree and your novel never gets published, you should still be able to love yourself. You should be able to find elements of yourself that you love that will be there no matter what. That will let you love yourself no matter what.'

He paused for a moment.

'If you can do this, then I think you'll go a long way towards conquering your depression.'

Over the next week or so, I battled to find things about myself that I liked. To find reasons that weren't related to "success" or "achievement" or anything of that nature was very hard for me, because they weren't ideas I'd ever considered before. All that had ever mattered to me was whether or not I was achieving my goals. If I was, or was on track to, then I loved myself. If I hadn't, or was not on track to, then I hated myself. The concept of loving myself regardless of whether or not I succeeded was completely foreign to me. But after a long time pondering, I finally managed to write the list that I included in the earlier chapter about learning how to love ourselves for healthy reasons. And when I focused on those healthy reasons, I could actually see that there really was a lot to love about me.

I actually am a good person, I remember thinking. *And this really is true, regardless of what my marks are at university or whether or not my novel ever gets published. These are the reasons why I can love myself, and whether I succeed or fail has nothing to do with it.*

This was such an empowering revelation, and once I'd made it, I took a huge step forward in conquering my depression.

If you too pin your self-worth to how well you achieve your goals, then I'd recommend writing a similar list of your own. Doing so, and having a revelation comparable to the one I had, doesn't

mean you stop striving to achieve your goals—rather, it just means that you stop hating yourself when you don't fulfil them.

Being perfectionistic can cause us to be neglectful

Because being perfectionistic leads us to be goal-orientated and pushes us to do our best in everything we do, it can sometimes lead us to neglect other things that matter—like our family or our health. For example, if we're always working late, then we may climb the corporate ladder quickly—but if we sacrifice exercising, then our health is going to suffer, and if we never socialise, then so will our relationships. Because of our hard work, we may well speed up the ranks—but is it really worth it if our partner leaves us? Or if we put on 60 pounds and develop diabetes?

One approach that's helped me keep things more in perspective is making a conscious effort to focus more on trying to be "happy" as opposed to trying to be "successful". They both certainly overlap to some degree, but I think the former is a vastly more well-rounded approach to life, and ever since adopting it, I've been much happier and healthier.

Perfectionism can lead us to procrastinate things or never get them finished

Doing things perfectly—or at least, to the very best of our ability—can be much more time consuming than just doing things well. And because us perfectionists are aware of this, we can often fall into the trap of putting off doing certain tasks altogether, because we can't find the time to do them "perfectly". Alternatively, we can spend so long trying to do something perfectly that we end up spending too

long on it or never getting it finished (I've found this to particularly be the case with projects that don't have a time deadline per se, such as writing my first novel or designing a website for my charity). In such cases, and in the cases where perfectionism leads us to procrastinate, I think it's important to remind ourselves that a job well done—albeit not a job perfectly done—is still better than a job not done at all.

Keep sharpening the good side of the sword, but try to blunt the bad side, too

We started this chapter by saying that perfectionism has a lot of positive aspects to it. This is definitely true, and for this reason, we certainly don't want to throw the baby out with the bath water just because it has the potential to lead to problems down the line. In my opinion, the best thing for us perfectionists to do is to just be mindful of the ways it may be hurting us, and if we find that it is, then take the necessary steps to correct it. On the whole, perfectionism is a great quality to have—we just have to make sure that it isn't triggering our depression and destroying our life.

Key takeaways from this chapter

1/ Being perfectionistic is a good thing, because it pushes us to strive for excellence and to reach our true potential. However, it also has its downfalls when it:

a) Leads us to measure our self-worth in terms of how "perfectly" we achieve our goals—which can lead us to feel worthless, inadequate, like a failure, and to hate ourselves;

b) Leads us to neglect some of life's most important aspects, such as our health and our relationships;

c) Leads us to procrastinate things or never quite finish them.

2/ We can prevent our perfectionistic tendencies from triggering our depression by:

a) Loving ourselves unconditionally.

b) Focusing on trying to be "happy" as opposed to being "successful".

c) Reminding ourselves that a job well done—albeit not a job perfectly done—is still better than a job not done at all.

CHAPTER 12
Common Cause of People's Depression #11:
Living an unhealthy lifestyle

"To keep the body in good health is a duty, otherwise we shall not be able to keep our mind strong and clear."
Buddha

Seemingly trivial things like eating well, sleeping well and exercising are easy things to forget about when we're trapped in the throes of depression. After all, when we're in that place, usually the last thing we want to do is go for a run. However, it's undeniable that if we do make the effort to live a healthy lifestyle, then it will significantly spur on our recovery. We'll talk about how we can do so in this chapter, with an emphasis on eating well, sleeping well and exercising frequently.

Eating well

The dietary guidelines for adults in Australia, as developed by the National Health and Medical Research Council, suggest that we should:

- Eat lots of vegetables, legumes and fruits;

- Eat plenty of cereals, including breads, rice, pasta and noodles (ideally of the wholegrain variety);
- Eat lean meat, fish, poultry and/or alternatives;
- Eat milks, yoghurts, cheeses and/or alternatives (ideally reduced fat substances, where possible);
- Drink lots of water;
- Limit saturated fat intake;
- Lean towards foods that are low in salt;
- Consume only moderate amounts of sugar;
- Minimise how much alcohol we drink.

Tools to help us eat healthily

Like we've said, when we suffer from depression, we're often so consumed with pain that we find it difficult to get anything done, including taking care with our diet and ensuring that we're eating healthily. However, this list of apps will make life easier:

1/ Swap It Don't Stop It: Developed by the Australian government, this app will help you make healthier food choices by showing you how to swap less nutritional foods for more nutritional substitutes, how to save calories, and much more. It's also possible to track your progress and set reminders to inform you when it's time to "make a swap".

2/ Fooducate: This app helps you make healthier choices when grocery shopping by illuminating the quality of calories in each item of food, and suggesting similar yet healthier alternatives.

3/ Loselt: If it's a weight loss plan you're after, this app can customise a plan for you that will suit your life. You can even start head-to-head, team- and group-based challenges with other people.

4/ HealthyOut: Tell this app your dietary restrictions and nutritional needs and it will suggest what you should eat at your restaurant of choice.

5/ ShopWell: Just by scanning the barcode, this app can tell you which foods at your supermarket meet your dietary needs based on your age, gender, health goals, diet needs, and ingredient and nutrition preferences.

6/ Zipongo: This app helps you eat healthily on the cheap, by letting you know about weekly sales at supermarkets in your area, and digital coupons that can save you money. It also contains lots of healthy eating tips and recipes.

7/ My Diet Coach: This app helps keep you motivated when you start a new weight loss plan by allowing you to upload photos and notes that inspire you, set reminders about what you want to eat and avoid, and make weight loss and fitness goals. You can even keep a food and exercise journal, and receive virtual prizes when you meet your targets.

8/ Calorie Counter and Tracker: Tell this app your age, gender and weight loss goals and it will help you reach them in your desired time frame. It also allows you to keep a food diary and keep track of how much exercise you're doing.

9/ Lifesum: If you prefer counting your kilojoule intake (as opposed to your calorie intake) then this app will help you do it. It also allows you to upload a "before healthy eating image" and helps you keep track of your weight so that you can reach your goals.

10/ Traffic Light Food Tracker: This app helps you compare packaged food products by entering the amount of salt, fat, saturated fat and sugar they contain per 100g. It will then display a traffic light for each nutrient: red indicating "high", yellow indicating "medium", and green indicating "low".

11/ MyFitnessPal: Enter your own recipes into this app and have MyFitnessPal calculate its nutritional information.

Are you drinking too much alcohol?

Like we've said, part of eating healthily involves limiting how much alcohol we drink. I know how tempting it can be to try and drown our depression in booze—being a recovered alcoholic, I've done it countless times myself. However, I can tell you from experience—and there are numerous studies to back me up—that drinking can significantly exacerbate our depression over time. Alcohol is a depressant after all—and, because of this, using it as an escape from our depression creates a devastatingly vicious cycle: we feel depressed, so we drink to feel better, which ultimately leads us to feel more depressed, which leads us to drink more, which leads us to feel even more depressed . . . and so the cycle goes, accelerating quicker and quicker since alcohol is also addictive. When we try to make ourselves feel better like this, we truly do become dogs endlessly chasing our tails.

As it always is with prevention, the less you drink, the better. However, below are some tell-tale signs that you may be hitting the bottle too hard.

1/ You go out with the intention of only having a couple of drinks, but you end up getting drunk;

2/ Your tolerance for alcohol has been increasing;

3/ You start to crave alcohol;

4/ Your drinking interferes with your day-to-day life because you're too drunk or hungover to get what you need to do done;

5/ You frequently go out with the objective of getting drunk;

6/ You continually find yourself in precarious situations while being under the influence;

7/ Your friends and family are hinting—or flat out telling you—that you're drinking too much;

8/ You've started drinking alone;

9/ Whenever something goes wrong or you're having a bad day, one of your first thoughts is, *I need a drink*;

10/ You don't know how to relax without alcohol;

11/ You aren't comfortable in social situations without alcohol;

12/ You plan your social and work calendar around alcohol;

13/ You hide the amount you drink from others;

14/ You've changed your drinking patterns to get drunk quicker (for example, by switching from wine or beer to spirits on the rocks);

15/ You've tried to quit drinking before but you haven't been able to.

If you found yourself relating to a lot of these scenarios, then chances are that your drinking is excessive enough that it's contributing to your depression (and quite possibly creating a number of other problems in your life, too). I'd strongly recommend significantly reducing how much alcohol you drink, and if that idea scares you, or if you've tried to cool it for a while and you haven't been able to, then it's worth seeking professional help.

What about drugs?

This almost goes without saying, but abusing illicit substances, just like drinking too much, will drastically undermine any attempt we make to recover from depression. Just like alcohol, it might help us escape our pain temporarily, but in the long run, it will keep us trapped in it forever.

Exercising

I know exercise is usually the last thing we feel like doing when we're suffering from depression, but if we give ourselves a push and do it, then we're going to enjoy the fruits of our labour. According to numerous studies, regular exercise can increase our level of brain serotonin and brain endorphins, both of which have "mood-lifting" properties. And, luckily for us, research also suggests that exercise doesn't have to be overly rigorous to be effective, with even a brisk walk said to make a noticeable difference.

Tools to help us exercise

This list of apps will help you create, strive for and reach your exercise goals:

1/ Cody: This app connects you with a fitness community where you can share and discover workouts complete with video, photo, and text instructions. Your friends are able to like and comment on your workout activity to help keep you motivated, and you can use the app's detailed statistical timeline to track your progress.

2/ Fitness Fast: This app provides instructions for a range of exercises targeting key muscles for pre-loaded or personally customised workouts. It also number-crunches a bunch of stats and other workout-related information, and offers a community forum for you to share and receive fitness information from others.

3/ Pact: This app uses financial incentives to encourage you to exercise. Each week, you'll pledge a set number of hours that you plan on exercising, and pledge a set amount of money that you'll pay up if you don't hit your target. If you do fulfil your pledge,

however, then you'll get paid! If you like the sound of this, then you can also use this app to enter into nutritional pacts, where you'll pay up if you don't achieve your healthy eating target, and get paid if you do.

4/ EveryMove: This rewards-based app lets you earn rewards points with different retailers when you exercise.

5/ Moves: This app calculates how many calories you're burning when you're running, walking or cycling.

6/ The Walk: Make exercise fun by turning a routine stroll into an incredible adventure! This app tracks how long and how far you've walked while you participate in games where your mission is to save the world. Before you begin your walk, you can choose an episode. The longer you walk, the more clues are revealed to help you in your quest.

7/ SecondsPro: This app allows you to create an extremely detailed, customised timer to help you complete your workouts. Even better, it can integrate with your I-pod, allowing you to assign playlists or tracks to individual timer intervals.

8/ Spring Moves: This app will scientifically create a personalised playlist for you based on your running rhythm!

9/ Strava Cycling: This app allows you to connect with other cyclists and challenge them to riding races. It also lets you and your friends support one another in each of your quests to achieve your cycling goals.

10/ Charity Miles: With this app, each mile you run, walk or cycle raises money for different non-profit organisations.

11/ Fitness Builder: This app gives you access to a library of over 5,600 exercise images and videos, and even gives you the option of picking a personal trainer's brain for advice.

12/ Daily Workouts: Perfect for busy people trying to squeeze in a workout on the fly, this app allows you to choose how long you want to exercise (10, 15, 20, 25 or 30 minutes) and which area of

your body you want to focus on. It then suggests an exercise for you to do, and shows you exactly how to do it.

Sleeping well

Depression is notorious for disrupting our sleep, but that doesn't change the fact that in order to recover, it really helps to get an average of seven or eight hours of sleep every night. To help you do so, I encourage you to use one or more of the following apps:

1/ SleepCycle: This app will analyse your sleep patterns and, within a desired interval, wake you up when you're in your lightest sleep phase so that you can start your day feeling more refreshed and energised. It can also map your sleep patterns over time to show how factors such as alcohol or exercise affect your rest.

2/ Sleep: This app plays soothing sounds, gentle lullabies and tranquil music to relax you in preparation for a good night of shuteye.

3/ Insomnia Cure: Containing hours of audio content and 40 pages of insomnia tips and learning tools, this app can finally help you get a good night's sleep.

4/ Nature Sounds Relax and Sleep: Whether it's a crackling campfire, songbirds, or the roar of the ocean surf that you find most relaxing, this app will help you unwind so that you fall asleep. All soundtracks are also accompanied by calming images.

5/ Long Deep Breathing: This app will teach you mindful breathing techniques that you can use to relax and help you fall asleep naturally.

6/ SleepBot: This app uses motion and sleep tracking capabilities to help you understand your sleep patterns, which can then help you make better decisions to improve your sleep habits. It's also got an

extensive database of sleep resources to teach you about good sleep hygiene, and allows you to keep track of your sleep history by date, sleep time, wake time, hours of sleep, or amount of sleep lost.

Key takeaways from this chapter

1/ In order to recover from depression, it's critical that we live a healthy lifestyle. This includes:

a) Eating well;
b) Laying off drugs and alcohol;
c) Exercising frequently;
d) Sleeping well.

2/ When we suffer from depression, living healthily can seem an overwhelming and sometimes impossible task. However, if we use a few of the countless apps that have been specifically developed to help us take better care of ourselves, then it will become a whole lot easier.

CHAPTER 13
Common Cause of People's Depression #12:

Having too many negative thoughts and not enough positive thoughts

"Positive thinking will let you do everything better than negative thinking will."
Zig Ziglar

It's no secret that when we have a negative thought, it can have a negative impact on our mood.

For example, thinking "nobody likes me" can cause us to feel sad.

Thinking that our partner is about to break up with us can make us feel scared and depressed.

Thinking that we're inadequate can make us feel jealous of other people.

Not only that, but studies have shown that when we have a negative thought, the left pre-frontal cortex part of our brain ("LPC") will then begin looking for examples in our lives that validate that negative thought.

For example, if we think the thought that "nobody likes me", then our LPC will automatically be steered towards finding more and more evidence to reinforce the belief that no-one likes us.

If we think that our partner's about to break up with us, then our LPC is going to go crazy looking for all sorts of signs to confirm the belief that we're about to get dumped.

And, if we think that we're inadequate, then our LPC is going to be focused on looking for more and more reasons to suggest that we're not as good as everybody else.

Due to the way our left pre-frontal cortexes work, negative thoughts set into motion a very poisonous cycle: the more negative thoughts we have, the harder our LPCs work to validate those thoughts . . . and the harder our LPCs work to validate those thoughts, the more negative thoughts we have . . . etcetera, etcetera, etcetera. As a result, one negative thought sets off a chain reaction of even stronger negative thoughts—negative thoughts that are so strong they can plunge us into depression.

Accordingly, in order to recover from depression, it's vital that we learn how to deal with those negative thoughts.

How can we manage our negative thoughts?

The following practices will help prevent us from experiencing negative thoughts, or help us deal with them when we do.

Challenge our negative thoughts

Our brains are great at playing tricks on us, often causing us to view our circumstances through pessimistic lenses. For this reason, in order to perceive our circumstances accurately and not allow our negative thoughts about those circumstances to trigger our depression, we need to challenge the rationality of our negative thoughts by asking ourselves the following questions:

- **What evidence is there to suggest that this thought is true? What evidence is there to suggest that it's false?** Remember how our left pre-frontal cortexes work? By looking for all the evidence they can to validate our negative thoughts? For this reason, when we take a step back and examine the evidence that is contrary to what our negative thoughts are telling us, we often end up with a much more accurate perception of our circumstances, and realise that they aren't as dire as we originally thought.
- **Is there a more positive, accurate way that I could be viewing this situation or circumstance?** In most cases, there usually is.
- **What would I tell my friend if they came to me saying that they're thinking this negatively about something**

in their life? Asking ourselves this question has the effect of distancing ourselves from our circumstances and looking at them from a different, more objective angle.

Avoid "black or white" thinking

When we think in terms of "black or white", everything is either good or bad, a success or a failure—there's nothing in between.

For example, *I'm not as well prepared for this exam as I'd like to be, so instead of acing it, I'm going to flunk.*

I know I don't look my best because I only had two minutes to get ready, so I must look terrible.

I said one silly little thing in my job interview today, so the whole thing was a complete disaster.

Thinking in this way can trigger our depression, because it leads us to conclude that just because something didn't—or isn't likely to—turn out perfectly, then it must be—or will be—an unmitigated catastrophe. However, when we think of our circumstances in such a rigid way, what we're not doing is acknowledging that in reality, there are many shades of grey, and that even though things may not turn out perfectly, they can still turn out OK.

Avoid making everything "about us"

Remember: if someone has a negative reaction to something we say or do, we can't jump to negative conclusions about ourselves. Doing so completely ignores the fact that we are only a part—and often only a very small part—of that person's world.

Avoid "filter thinking"

"Filter thinking" is when we filter out all the praise that is coming our way and instead only listen to the criticism. For example, our university professor returns our essay—it gets 90% and receives lots of positive feedback, but our professor also offers some constructive criticism and suggestions for improvement—however, instead of focusing on all the good things we did, we completely block them out, and only focus on what we didn't do well. As a result, we conclude that we're not very clever, and begin to feel depressed.

To avoid "filter thinking", it helps to get a piece of paper and make two columns—one for the positive feedback we received, and one for the not-so-positive feedback. Then, we want to write down all the feedback we received in their respective columns. If we're thinking with a filter, we'll soon realise that we're blowing the negative feedback we received out of proportion.

Minimise the time we spend doing things that trigger negative thoughts

We can reduce the number of negative thoughts we have by figuring out what causes us to think negative thoughts, and then making a determined effort to minimise—and ideally eliminate—the time we spend doing such things.

For example, I find the news very negative, because in Australia at least, most of what's shown on the news is bad news. I'm not denying that bad things happen in the world, but beautiful, miraculous, unbelievably positive things occur every day as well—and yet for some reason, it's usually only the tragedies that hit the air. Accordingly, I find the news to be a skewed portrayal of life, and in the vast majority of cases, anything but uplifting.

Consequently, watching the news leads me to have negative thoughts. Whenever I used to watch it, I'd find myself thinking,

Wow, there really are a lot of bad things happening in the world! It's all just one heartbreaking incident after another. How come nothing good ever happens?

And when I had these thoughts, my LPC would then look to further validate them by finding all the evidence it could to support their premise. Accordingly, I'd find myself zeroing in on all the sad and devastating things that were happening in the world, and completely ignoring all the good things that were simultaneously occurring. As a result, my mood would nosedive.

For this reason, part of my recovery from depression involved—as silly and as trivial as it sounds—me deciding to quit watching the news. And ever since I've stopped doing so, I've felt a whole lot better.

In terms of *how* we can figure out what's causing us to think negative thoughts, we can keep a thought diary. Similar in concept to keeping a mood diary, taking note of all the things that cause us to think negative thoughts can help us figure out what we're doing that is causing us to think so negatively. After we've pinpointed those causes, we can then take steps to minimise the time we spend on them.

Avoid trying to predict the future

Sometimes when something hasn't worked out well in the past, we convince ourselves that that something's destined never to work out in the future as well. But if we learn everything we can from the experience the first time something goes awry, then we'll be much more prepared the next time to ensure a better result. Primarily for this reason, history does not have to repeat itself. If we can remember this, and learn to take things on a case-by-case basis, then

we can eliminate a lot of our negative thinking, and be all the happier for it.

Distinguish our thoughts from reality

Instead of saying, for example, "no-one likes me" and accepting it as reality, it can help to instead say, "I'm having the thought that no-one likes me". Although this may seem like a trivial distinction, doing this gives us distance from our thoughts, and helps us realise that that's all they are—thoughts—as opposed to cold, hard, irrefutable facts.

Avoid toxic people

Toxic people certainly have the power to cause us to think negative thoughts, and the sooner we distance ourselves from them, the less negatively we'll think.

Do our minds work the "other way", too?

When I first learned about how our negative thoughts affect our mood and about the power of our LPCs to contribute to our depression by looking for evidence to verify our negative thoughts, I immediately wondered if our brains also worked the "other way", too.

If I have a positive *thought,* I remember thinking, *then does that mean that our LPCs will look for evidence to validate that thought too, and as a result, contribute to putting us in a positive mood?*

And the answer, I was pleased to find out, is yes! That's exactly how our LPCs work!

For example, when we have a positive thought like "my life is good", our LPCs will get to work trying to find all the evidence they can to validate the notion that we have a really good life. As a result, we're likely to find ourselves in a pleasant mood, because we're going to be highly mindful of and focused on all the reasons why we have a good life—as opposed to the reasons that lead us to believe that our life isn't so good.

For this reason, in order to recover from depression and start living the happy life we want, it's critical that we not only take steps to minimise how many negative thoughts we have, but that we also take steps to *maximise* how many *positive* thoughts we have.

What can we do to have more positive thoughts?

Below is a list of things we can do to have more positive thoughts. You'll notice that we've talked about many of them in different contexts before.

- **Spend more time outdoors.** This may sound frivolous, but exposure to the sun increases the amount of serotonin (AKA the "happy chemical") in our brain.
- **Maximise the time we spend doing things we enjoy.**
- **Surround ourselves with the "right" people for us.**
- **Practice gratitude.**
- **Live healthily—i.e. eat well, sleep well and exercise frequently.**

Key takeaways from this chapter

1/ Our thoughts control our moods, and due to the way the left pre-frontal cortex part of our brain works, one negative thought can set off a chain reaction of even stronger negative thoughts, which can have the power to trigger our depression.

2/ We can reduce or eliminate our negative thoughts by challenging their validity, avoiding "black or white" thinking, not making everything "about us", avoiding "filter thinking", minimising the time we spend doing things that trigger negative thoughts, reminding ourselves that the future doesn't have to be the same as the past, distinguishing our thoughts from reality, and avoiding toxic people.

3/ We can have more positive thoughts by spending more time in the sun, reading positive affirmations, maximising the time we spend doing things we enjoy, surrounding ourselves with the "right" people for us, practising gratitude, and exercising.

CHAPTER 14
Common Cause of People's Depression #13:
Worrying

"Worry does not take away tomorrow's troubles. Instead, it takes away today's joy."

When I suffered from depression, this was something that I used to do all the time. Whenever I had an exam at university for example, I remember worrying that I wouldn't study for something that would surprisingly be on the test, and that I'd end up doing badly as a result; I'd worry that I'd misread the exam details and turn up to the wrong room; or, I'd worry that I'd oversleep my alarm and not turn up at all. Worrying can be beneficial when it galvanises us to do what's necessary to solve a problem, but if we're obsessing over "what-ifs" and worst-case scenarios like so, then it can significantly trigger our depression.

What can we do to stop worrying so much?

What my psychologist taught me is that when we find ourselves worrying, the first thing we want to do is stop and take a few minutes

to *dissect* our worry. Specifically, we want to ask ourselves the following question:

Is there something I can do to fix the problem that's troubling me? Or, is what I'm worrying about out of my control?

Now, if there's something we can do to fix the problem that's troubling us, then we need to turn our attention to doing everything we can to fix it.

However, if we find that we're worrying about something that is out of our control, then it means that our worrying is unproductive, and is doing nothing more than stressing us out and igniting our depression. For this reason, it's vital that we stop worrying about whatever we're worrying about. The following suggestions can help us do this.

Challenge our worry

Similar to when we're thinking negatively, when we're jumping to conclusions, fretting over "what-ifs" and going crazy thinking about all the worst possible scenarios that could ever take place, what we're usually doing is viewing our circumstances in a much darker light than they really are. Such pessimistic thinking can often come very naturally to us, but in order to prevent our worry from destroying our lives, we need to retrain our brains to think about our circumstances more realistically—i.e. in their proper, brighter light.

In order to do this, we need to start by zeroing in on our worrying thought. Then, instead of accepting it as gospel, we must challenge its validity by asking the following questions (a few of which will sound familiar):

- **What evidence is there to suggest that this thought is true? What evidence is there to suggest that it's false?**

- **Is there a more positive, accurate way that I could be viewing this situation or circumstance?**

- **Realistically, what is the probably that what I'm stressing out about will actually take place?** Studies indicate that 85% of what we worry about never happens. In all likelihood, what we're worrying about is much less likely to occur than we think.

- **If what I'm stressing out about does take place, does it mean that my life is over? Or, will I be able to cope with it and recover in time?** Studies also indicate that even if what we're worrying about does occur, then 80% of us handle it better than we originally thought we would. We need to give ourselves credit for being stronger than we think, and acknowledge that even if something bad does unfortunately take place, that we have the strength to survive it and overcome it in time.

- **What would I tell my friend if they came to me saying that they're worrying about this problem?** When I ask myself this question, most of the time I envision myself saying to my friend, "just try to relax . . . everything is going to be OK". And when I imagine myself saying this, I realise that my worrying is nothing more than over-reacting, and then I'm able to let it go.

Tolerate uncertainty

After I'd quit Commerce/Law to pursue my dream of becoming an author, there were times when I'd worry that my novel would never get published and that instead of achieving my dream, I'd wind up a broke, lonely, miserable old man. But then my psychologist offered me some advice that has stuck with me ever since.

'I think you need to focus more on the journey you're on, and less on the end outcome,' he said one day when I expressed my concerns to him. 'It's going to be a while before your novel is completely finished and ready to try and publish, so there's no need to think about what's going to happen then until the moment's upon you. Right now, just enjoy yourself. After all, you're writing full-time—right now, you're *already* living your dream! Experience it to the full. Be wholly present in the moment. Enjoy it for what it is instead of fretting about whether or not you'll get published and what may or may not happen if you don't. Whenever you do stress about all that, you're only taking away from your enjoyment of this exciting journey that you're embarking upon. Later on, if you do end up getting rejected by every agent and publisher in the business, you can worry. But right now—just forget about it.'

Accordingly, one of the most important steps I took in reducing how much I worried was learning to accept and tolerate uncertainty. Once I'd accepted that it was an inherent part of my life and detrimental to my happiness to worry about, I naturally started focusing more on enjoying the present, and stopped stressing so much about "what-ifs" and worst-case scenarios.

Keep a worry diary

Similar in concept to keeping a mood- or a thoughts diary, taking note of all the things that cause us to worry over time can help us figure out the sources of our worry. We can then take steps to eliminate those sources, and thus become much more at peace with the world.

Keep repeating what we're worried about until we accept it

If we repeat something that we're worried about again and again and again, we'll gradually come to accept that something as a possibility that may occur, and in the course of doing so, it will begin to lose its ability to worry us. For example, if I'd have kept saying to myself, "my novel may never get published, my novel may never get published", then such a notion would have eventually lost its power to scare me.

Write down what we're worrying about

Studies suggest that writing down our worries can help us come to terms with them, and similar to the way repeating them over and over again does, rob them of their power to worry us.

Meditation

Studies indicate that meditating can lower our anxiety levels and greatly reduce how much we worry.

Distract ourselves by doing something enjoyable

If we can lose ourselves in something pleasurable, then we'll be too busy having fun to worry about whatever it is that we shouldn't be worried about.

Exercise

Getting our heart rate up is a great way to relieve our stress and forget about our problems for a while.

Key takeaways from this chapter

1/ When we catch ourselves worrying, we need to stop and ask ourselves the question: *Is there something I can do to fix the problem that's troubling me? Or, is what I'm worrying about out of my control?* If there's something we can do to fix it, then we should try to fix it. However, if there's nothing we can do, then our worrying is unproductive, and it's vital to our mental health that we cease doing so.

2/ We can stop worrying about things that are out of our control by challenging our worry, tolerating uncertainty, keeping a worry diary, keep repeating what we're worrying about until we accept it, writing down what we're worrying about, meditating, distracting ourselves by doing something enjoyable, and exercising.

CHAPTER 15
Common Cause of People's Depression #14:
Struggling to trust someone again after we've been hurt in love

"We're never so vulnerable as when we trust someone—but paradoxically, if we cannot trust, neither can we find love or joy."
Walter Anderson

Have you ever been through one of those terrible relationships or break-ups that leave you doubting whether or not you'll ever be able to trust someone again?

I have. And so have countless other people.

In fact, fear of trusting someone again is such a common reaction to being hurt in love that it has its own name: *pistanthrophobia*.

As any of us who've been there will agree, it's an extremely difficult thing to get over. However, if we want to be in a happy, healthy relationship again, then we do need to overcome it. The four suggestions below helped me, and if pistanthrophobia is triggering your depression, then I think they'll also help you get past some of the things that are holding you back from a brighter future.

Don't assume the future will be the same as the past

As you know, my first proper relationship ended when I found out that my girlfriend was cheating on me with one of my best mates; then afterwards—perhaps to get back at me for breaking up with her—I heard that she'd been spreading the (extremely false) rumour that I'd raped her. I was shattered. Combined with some of the other things that were taking place in my life at the time, the experience plunged me into a crippling and near fatal depression, and my ability to trust another girl was destroyed.

Over the next few years, I brought my pistanthrophobia with me on every date I went on, and suffice it to say, there weren't a lot of second dates. My inability to trust another girl was ruining any chance I had of being in a functional relationship, and I wondered if I'd ever be able to overcome it and make things work with a woman.

Eventually however, I started seeing a therapist for my depression. Everything that happened with my ex inevitably came up, and my psychologist gave me a piece of advice that helped me immensely:

Don't cast dispersions on the entire female population because of one bad experience with one bad girl.

I think casting such dispersions is the root cause of the vast majority of people's pistanthrophobia; because we've been hurt by one person—or in some cases, a number of people—we become conditioned to believing that the next person will hurt us too. But projecting this assumption onto the next person isn't being fair. Unless that person has done something to make us wary of trusting them, then they deserve to be given an open-minded chance. It's important that we start each relationship with a clean slate, and not let it be poisoned by our past.

Learn from the past: what were the warning signs that our ex was untrustworthy?

In my case, my ex would constantly break promises, lie, say one thing then do something else, and continuously do things that she knew would bother me. With the benefit of hindsight, it's not surprising that she ended up seriously hurting me. People who have certain self-centred, manipulative and malicious traits are not worthy of our trust. If we can learn from our past relationships to identify such traits and the types of people who aren't to be trusted, then we'll be better at picking a lover the next time around—and knowing that we're wiser and more likely to pick a better lover will make us less scared of getting hurt.

Learn from the past: what were the things that we could have done differently?

The way my ex used to look at my mate, the amount they used to talk to each other on the phone, the amount of time they'd always spend together . . . I was always suspicious that something was going on. But whenever I'd bring it up with her, she'd always stress that they were just friends, and feeling guilty for raising it, I'd let the matter drop—even though my gut was telling me that something wasn't right. In the end of course, I ended up being correct.

The key lesson I learned from this was to trust my instincts. Where there's smoke there's often fire, so if something seems off to us, then it probably is. Part of the lesson I learned is that my girlfriend should have addressed my fears and not dismissed them. As a result of learning this lesson, I now have confidence in myself that should a similar situation present itself, I won't make the same mistake. And once we trust ourselves to be able to make better

decisions in the future, it becomes much easier to trust somebody else.

Give ourselves time to heal

After a difficult break-up, I think it's extremely helpful to take a timeout from dating and try to grow in our pain. I personally rushed back into things when in hindsight I wasn't ready, and all it did was lead to more failed relationships, which led to more heartache, which led to more pistanthrophobia, which led to more failed relationships, which led to more heartache, which led to more pistanthrophobia . . . etcetera, etcetera, etcetera. Instead, I think it's better to learn everything we can from our previous relationships, and work to arrive at a place where we feel that if we were to meet someone else that we're interested in, we'd be able to start fresh. Once we've done that, then we're ready to start dating again.

The best revenge is living well

As the saying goes, once we're bitten, we're twice shy. The natural intention is to put up barriers around us and try to protect ourselves by refusing to open up and trust anyone again. But if we do that, we could miss out on the joy of spending our lives with someone great. And we should try our damnedest not to let that happen. An ex's deceitfulness does not have to have a permanent impact on our ability to trust another person, and it doesn't have to destroy our future relationships.

After all, our ex has already hurt us enough. We don't want to give them the power to hurt us anymore.

Key takeaways from this chapter

1/ Fear of trusting someone again can be very difficult for us to recover from, but if we want to be in a happy, healthy relationship again, then we *do* need to overcome it.

2/ The four suggestions that helped me recover from my pistanthrophobia were:

a) Not making the assumption that the future will be the same as the past;

b) Understanding the warning signs that my ex was untrustworthy, which will protect me in the future by helping me recognise similar signs in another person who may also be untrustworthy;

c) Learning what I can do differently to prevent a similar heartbreak from occurring in the future;

d) Giving myself time to heal from my pain.

CHAPTER 16
What steps can we take to learn how to deal with any causes of our depression that weren't discussed in this book?

"An investment in knowledge always pays the best interest"

Benjamin Franklin

In chapters 2-15, we covered a bunch of particularly common causes of people's depression and talked about how we can deal with them. But of course, we didn't cover *every* possible cause, because unfortunately, there are just too many of them. If one or more of the causes of your depression weren't analysed in this book, then I recommend taking the following steps to learn how to deal with them. In fact, I strongly encourage you to take the following steps anyway, even if *all* the causes of your depression were covered in this book, because doing so will give you additional insight and help you deal with them at an even quicker rate.

See a therapist

Like we said way back in chapter 1, this is part of a therapist's job— —to teach us how to deal with the underlying causes of our

depression. The way I always thought of it was like this: a person with depression has a broken brain, and they need therapy to mend it—in the same way that a person with a broken leg needs surgery to fix it. And, in the same way that a broken leg will never heal without surgery—or, at the very best, not heal properly—a broken brain will never heal properly—or at all—without therapy. Seeing a therapist gave me my life back, and I really, really recommend that you see one too.

Read self-help books

Another thing we can do is read self-help books about how to recover from depression. The best ones are written by some of the most respected psychologists and psychiatrists in the world, and can be immensely valuable resources—particularly if we don't have access to one-to-one therapy. Books I recommend in particular are:

- *Feeling Good* by Dr David D Burns;
- *Authentic Happiness* by Dr Martin E. P. Seligman;
- *The Mindful Way Through Depression* by Mark Williams, John Teasdale, Zindel Segal and John Kabat-Zinn.

Of course, there are also self-help books written about specific causes of depression. Whether it's a lack of self-esteem that's at the root of your depression, a fear of intimacy, difficulty being assertive or something else, you can be sure that there's been a book written on the topic by a renowned psychologist or psychiatrist that you can find on Amazon.

Do online therapy . . . for free!

Given that many people with depression don't have access to private therapy, the availability of free online therapy programs is something that isn't publicised anywhere near enough. There are some great programs out there run by some of the best universities in the world, and building this type of therapy into our day is likely to do wonders over time. The one I recommend using is MoodGYM, which is run by the prestigious Australian National University. To quote their website:

MoodGYM is an innovative, interactive web program designed to prevent depression. It consists of five modules: an interactive game, anxiety and depression assessments, downloadable relaxation audio, a workbook and feedback assessment.

Using flashed diagrams and online exercises, MoodGYM teaches the principles of cognitive behavioural therapy—a proven treatment for depression. It also demonstrates the relationship between thoughts and emotions, and works through dealing with stress and relationship break-ups, as well as teaching relaxation and meditation techniques.

The Australian National University has also recently brought out E-couch, their newest online program for preventing and coping with depression, generalised anxiety disorder, and social anxiety disorder. Like MoodGYM, it's also free.

A final note on dealing with the causes of our depression

After reading the last hundred or so pages of this book, I hope you can see how vital it is to your recovery to learn how to deal with the causes of your depression.

And it really is vital, because here's the reality:

Most of our triggers will never go away.

Let's take my perfectionism as an example. For the rest of my life, there are going to be times when I don't achieve a goal that I set out to achieve. And, if I'd never learned how deal with this cause of my depression, then I'd always feel depressed every time I didn't achieve one of my goals. But since I now know how to deal with it——along with the other causes of my depression—I have recovered from my illness, and now live a very happy, healthy life.

If we can learn how to deal with all of the causes of our depression so that they no longer cause us to feel depressed, then we can recover from depression. But if we don't learn how to deal with them, the sad reality is that we'll probably battle depression for the rest of our lives.

Key takeaways from this chapter

1/ Three things we can do to learn how to deal with the causes of our depression that haven't been covered in this book include:

a) Seeing a therapist;

b) Reading self-help books;

c) Doing free online therapy at MoodGym.

2/ If we learn how to deal with the underlying causes of our depression, then we can recover. However if we don't, then we'll probably suffer from depression for the rest of our lives.

Step 3: Learning how to handle a relapse

CHAPTER 17

"Part of recovery is relapse. I dust myself off and move forward again."

Steven Adler

Like we've been saying throughout this book, when we're suffering from depression, we want to work through the first two steps we outlined—i.e. we want to figure out what's causing our depression (Step 1), and then we want to figure out how to deal with the underlying causes of our depression so that they no longer cause us to feel depressed (Step 2). Once we've done this, we'll recover from that particular episode of depression. However, in the future, we may experience a relapse.

For many people, experiencing a relapse is a huge cause for concern. It used to be for me, too.

How the hell could I feel so good, feel so certain that I'd conquered my demons, only to feel depressed again a short while later? I used to think.

And then came the most terrifying thought that a person with depression can possibly have:

Will I always feel this way? Is this just the way I am? Will I forever be condemned to a life of insufferable pain and despair?

I get it. However, what I eventually realised is that what having a relapse means is that at the point in time we're having one, we're not yet able to deal with the causes of our depression to an extent so masterful as to prevent them from depressing us.

That's such an important point that I'm going to say it again.

What having a relapse means is that at the point in time we're having one, we're not yet able to deal with the causes of our depression to an extent so masterful as to prevent them from depressing us.

So what do we do then?

When we experience a relapse, then instead of panicking, we want to repeat steps one and two—i.e. we want to put more work into understanding what is causing that particular bout of depression, and then put more work into learning how to deal with that cause so that it no longer has the power to trigger our depression.

We can repeat steps one and two by, for example:

- Going back and re-reading the relevant chapters in this book to better deal with the causes of our depression;
- Going back to see our therapist if we've stopped, or start seeing them more regularly if we haven't;
- Going back to our doctor to see if there's a more effective medication and/or dosage we could be taking.

I'm telling you, if you repeat steps one and two every time you experience a relapse, then your relapses will gradually become less and less intense, and fewer and farther between—and eventually, you can stop having relapses altogether.

To quote a metaphor from my memoir *Depression is a Liar*:

> *It's as if there's a fortress surrounding our brains that's there to protect us from getting depressed, and every time we repeat steps one and two, another armed guard gets posted outside it. If depression's army still gets*

through from time to time, then it just means there aren't enough guards defending it yet. But if we keep repeating steps one and two, we will eventually have so many guards protecting us that depression's army will be shut out for good. It'll have no way of getting through.

And it's because of this exact reason that if you follow this three step approach, you really can recover from depression eventually. It will be extremely difficult, because you will have to be proactive when you feel exhausted, you will have to fight when you feel like giving up, and you will have to remain hopeful when depression is doing everything in its power to break your will. But if you follow this three step process, you can get there in the end, because as I like to say, while it is hard for a person to beat depression, it's even harder for depression to beat a person who never gives up.

OTHER BOOKS BY DANNY BAKER

Depression is a Liar (2013)

A #1 international mental health bestseller

After graduating from high school at the top of his year and accepting a scholarship to study Commerce/Law at Sydney University, Danny Baker seemed destined to become a wealthy investment banker or management consultant, live the high life and retire young. But a spiralling descent into depression shattered his world, and for the next four years, the only thing Baker seemed destined for was a life of never-ending misery. Eventually, however, he managed to recover, and these days, is happy, healthy and absolutely loves his life – albeit a life that's far, far removed from what he once thought it would be.

Written almost two years after his last depressive episode, *Depression is a Liar* is a nakedly honest, gritty account of Baker's struggle and eventual triumph over his illness. In his own words:

"I wanted to tell my story so that people with depression could realise that they're not alone. Of course, I also wanted to share the lessons I learned on the long, rocky, winding road that eventually led to recovery – particularly with regards to relationships; substance abuse; choosing a fulfilling career path; perfectionism; seeking professional help; and perhaps most importantly, having a positive, healthy attitude towards depression that enables recovery. Above all else, however, I wrote this memoir to give sufferers hope,

and to show them that no matter how much they're struggling, that recovery is always, always possible."

I Will Not Kill Myself, Olivia (2015)

An Amazon UK Top 100 bestseller

Like most young adults, Jimmy Wharton is trying to carve out a happy, successful life for himself. It's hard enough to do under any circumstances, but when he starts suffering from depression, becoming the person he wants to be feels overwhelmingly unachievable, as his illness seems destined to shatter his world.

Olivia, Jimmy's high school sweetheart and long-term girlfriend, initially tries to support him in every way she can. But as Jimmy spirals downwards, their relationship begins to break at the seams, and they are forced to face the devastating reality that as strong as they know their love is, the force of Jimmy's depression could be even stronger.

Set against the backdrop of Sydney's iconic Manly Beach, *I Will Not Kill Myself, Olivia* is a tale about the intoxicating, heartbreaking, unforgettable experience of first love; about all the mistakes we make on the road to adulthood; and about an illness that afflicts 350 million people worldwide.

ABOUT THE AUTHOR

Danny Baker was born and raised in Sydney, Australia. In 2007 he took a scholarship to study commerce/law at Sydney University before trading in his textbooks in 2012 to pursue his dream of becoming an author. At the time of writing, he's published three books: *This Is How You Recover From Depression;* the Amazon UK Top 100 bestseller *I Will Not Kill Myself, Olivia* – which is a story about a love triangle involving a guy, a girl and depression; and the #1 international mental health bestseller *Depression is a Liar* – which recounts Danny's struggle and eventual triumph over depression.

To find out more about Danny's books or to get in touch, visit his website at www.dannybakerwrites.com.